Weight Perfect
THIRD EDITION

BY MARY O'BRIEN, M.D.

©2019   INR Books   Concord, California

Weight Perfect
THIRD EDITION

INSTITUTE FOR NATURAL RESOURCES (INR)
P.O. Box 5757
Concord, CA 94524-0757
USA

tel: 925-609-2820
fax: 925-363-7798
info@biocorp.com

AUTHOR
Mary O'Brien, M.D.

About The Author

Dr. Mary O'Brien, M.D. is board-certified in internal medicine and geriatrics and has served on the medical school faculties of Georgetown University and the University of North Carolina. She is also a board-certified Physician Nutrition Specialist.

Special Thanks

Contributing Writers
Craig Freudenrich, Ph.D.
Barbara Sternberg, Ph.D.
Roxanne Nelson, R.N.
Amy Erickson
Harmony Raylen Abejuela

Contributing Editors
Richard S. Colman, Ph.D.
Holly Stevens
Linda Hudson

Dedication

This book is dedicated to those who have suffered through devastating natural disasters and the selfless rescue and relief workers who help. They teach us what really matters in life.

Mary O'Brien, M.D.

About INR (INSTITUTE FOR NATURAL RESOURCES)

INR is an non-profit organization that provides health care professionals with the latest scientific and clinical information. INR's live seminars and home-study courses are designed to help health professionals provide better care for their patients. INR operates nationwide in the United States as well as internationally.

Table of Contents

CHAPTER 1   8
why weight matters

CHAPTER 2   44
the food-sleep connection: insomnia & obesity

CHAPTER 3   72
medical conditions & weight gain

CHAPTER 4   104
fad diets & popular weight loss plans: which ones work?

CHAPTER 5   136
emotions & overeating: how to stop the cycle

CHAPTER 6   166
controlling cravings

CHAPTER 7   192
obesity medications

CHAPTER 8   214
devices & surgery: the last options

CHAPTER 9   232
the genetic puzzle: providing clues for obesity treatment

CHAPTER 10   248
fit for life

CHAPTER 11   276
weight perfect: optimal weight for life

REFERENCES   305

GLOSSARY   319

Chapter 1

why weight matters

"Eat...to live, and do not live to eat."

~ William Penn, 1693

"Being obese is like being 20 years older than
you really are. It does more damage to your
quality of life, causes more chronic medical
conditions, and incurs more healthcare
expenditures than either smoking or
alcohol abuse."

~ Roland Sturm, economist, RAND
Corporation

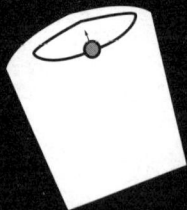

Obesity in the U.S. is now at epidemic proportions. As Americans have increased their girth, rates of obesity-related illness such as heart disease and diabetes have also skyrocketed. Children and teenagers are joining the ranks of the overweight and obese in greater numbers too. And they're at much higher risk than ever before for obesity-related diseases.

There are many reasons for the obesity epidemic, including greater availability of junk foods, declining activity levels, and a commuter lifestyle that emphasizes meals that are convenient, rather than nutritious. But that's not to say that being overweight is inevitable. With some common sense tips and simple lifestyle changes we'll show you, you'll find it's possible to lose weight—and lose those pounds for good.

If you can successfully lose weight and keep it off, you'll be more likely to avoid illnesses such as cancer, kidney disease, heart disease, arthritis, and even cataracts. You'll also have a much better chance of adding years to your life, and enjoying those years more fully. Whether you're age 18 or 85, it's never a bad time to dedicate yourself to lasting weight loss, and to reap the rewards of a healthy lifestyle.

OBESITY: A WORLDWIDE EPIDEMIC

If you worry about your weight, you are not alone. More than 105 million adults in the U.S. are overweight or obese. Despite the fitness craze of the last 30 years and the popularity of diets ranging from Atkins to Weight Watchers, we continue to pack on the pounds. The result is that overweight and obesity now tops the list of major medical problems in the U.S.

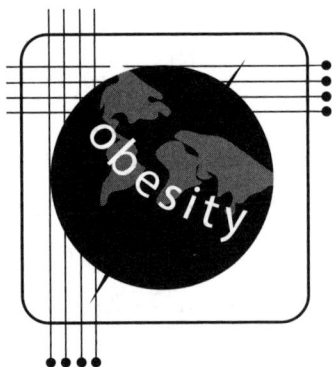

Obesity is now considered to be a health pandemic—an epidemic that touches many nations around the world, including developing and industrialized countries such as the United States. According to the World Health Organization (WHO), there are 1.1 billion overweight people on our planet, as well as 300 million adults classified as obese.

Being overweight or obese can lead to increased risk of chronic conditions including diabetes, heart disease, arthritis, cancer, and even depression. But the good news is that losing extra pounds—even 10% of your body weight—can significantly reduce these health risks, and may even help you live longer.

Nearly two thirds of all adults in the U.S. are either overweight or obese. The percentage of overweight children and adolescents has more than doubled since the early 1970s, and it is estimated that 31% of juveniles are carrying excess body fat. These extra pounds have consequences. Those who tip the scales during their teen years have a 70% chance of becoming overweight or obese adults.

The percentage of overweight children and adolescents has more than doubled since the early 1970s...

Modifiable behavioral risk factors—habits and lifestyles that we have control over are the leading causes of mortality. Our eating habits and couch-potato lifestyle are now causing almost as many deaths as smoking.

Maintaining a healthy weight is crucial for our overall health, as well as our lifespan. And, despite what many diet books promise, there is no magic formula for weight loss. Losing weight successfully means choosing to change the lifestyle habits that put on the pounds in the first place: spending more time engaged in physical activity, making wiser dietary choices, and finding ways to comfort and reward ourselves without resorting to too many hot fudge sundaes and pepperoni pizzas.

WHY ARE WE GAINING SO MUCH WEIGHT?

The encroachment of obesity on our society as a whole has become increasingly troubling. In a relatively short time, we have transformed ourselves from a relatively fit and trim population into one that is bursting at the seams.

Why has obesity suddenly become so prevalent? That's a crucial question. While hereditary factors may account for 30% or more of obesity cases, it would be difficult to chalk it all up to genetics.

After all, our genes haven't changed over the course of a few decades.

Most experts agree that the primary causes of obesity are a sedentary lifestyle and a diet rich in high-calorie food. If you consume more calories than you expend, you will eventually gain weight. For some people, however, it is not that simple.

Many factors contribute to excess weight gain. Besides our genes, socioeconomic level, environmental and cultural influences, metabolic effects, and behavioral issues all influence the tendency to gain weight. Some of us can wolf down half a pint of ice cream and not gain an ounce, while others struggle with the "battle of the bulge" for the better part of their lives. Most of us fall somewhere in between when it comes to controlling our weight.

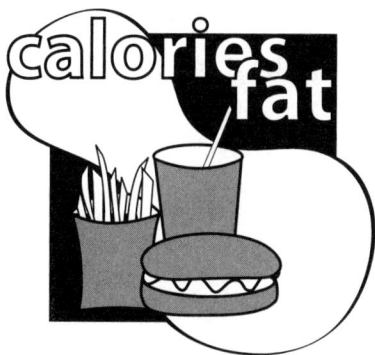

Many factors contribute to weight gain. Large portions, frequent snacking, sugar-laden beverages, stress eating, and sedentary living all play a role.

Eating out on a frequent basis is also associated with weight gain. Busy lifestyles have made dining out more popular. In fact, Americans spend an estimated 50% of their food budgets on meals eaten outside of their homes. On average, commercially prepared food is less nutritious and often higher in fat and lower in nutrients than a meal prepared in our own kitchens.

Americans spend an estimated 50% of their food budgets on meals eaten outside of their homes.

Over the past 30 years, portion sizes in restaurants have also mushroomed. It is impossible to ignore the "supersizing" that has become so commonplace. Half a century ago, a serving of french fries at a fast food outlet was about 2 ounces, but today it is two to three times that size. The original burger and fries from McDonald's, along with a 12-ounce serving of Coke, totaled 590 calories. Compare that to today's version: A supersize Quarter Pounder with Cheese, supersize fries, and supersize Coke adds up to a whopping 1,550 calories. Even the simple bagel has doubled or even tripled in size, from 2 to 3 ounces a few decades ago, to 4 to 7 ounces now.

Unfortunately, sit-down restaurants are also filling our plates with more food than ever before. And research shows that portion size directly influences how much you eat. If you are served more, you eat more.

Desserts, pastries, and soft drinks head the list of foods that contribute the most calories to the typical American diet. Vegetables and fruits, on the other hand, barely make an appearance. High in nutrition and fiber, and low in calories and fat, they account for only 10% of calories in the average diet.

Perhaps most worrisome is the impact of fast food on children. Their consumption of fast food has increased five-fold over the past 30 years. Nearly one third of all youngsters from age 4 to 19 have a daily fast food meal, which packs on about six extra pounds a year. Children who frequently dine at fast food eateries eat more fat and sugar, and fewer fruits and non-starchy vegetables than other children.

Another piece in the obesity puzzle may be the increasing consumption of high-fructose corn syrup (HFCS) as a sweetener in foods and drinks. Made from hydrolyzed cornstarch, HFCS is very sweet and inexpensive. It is added to an enormous assortment of items, including sodas, juice, cookies, yogurt, ketchup, cereals, and soup. HFCS use rose more than 1,000% between 1970 and 1990, and now accounts for over 40% of caloried sweeteners that are added to foods and drinks, according to a study published in the *American Journal of Clinical Nutrition*.

Animal models show that fructose consumption correlates with insulin resistance, impaired glucose tolerance, hypertension, and increased triglyceride levels The data on the effects of HFCS in humans is not as clear, but many researchers believe this sweetener is adding to our obesity woes.

NOT ENOUGH EXERCISE

Another problem that contributes to obesity in our society is widespread physical inactivity, especially among children. America has become a nation of couch potatoes.

One in four children nationwide have no physical education at all. And almost half of young people between 12 and 21 do not participate in any regular vigorous physical activity. Hours on end spent glued to assorted devices, games, and social media sites have clearly had negative consequences on many levels.

Many of us spend nine hours sitting at a desk, get in the car to drive home, pick up dinner along the way, and then spend the evening in front of the television set or a smartphone. Suburban neighborhoods frequently discourage physical exercise: They lack sidewalks, play areas for children, access to public transportation, or shopping within walking distance. Recreational facilities such as parks and community centers may be far away or non-existent.

We take elevators instead of the stairs, and indeed, many office buildings lock the stairwells, reserving them for emergencies. Children are often driven to school or arrive by school bus, have no physical activity during the course of the school day, then come home and sit in front of their devices.

Many risk factors play a role in the national weight gain.

Some of us are more genetically predisposed to gain weight. Genetic variations help explain why some individuals are prone to weight gain, and find it difficult to slim down, while others rarely gain. Obesity appears to run in families, and it can be caused by a particular gene, a combination of genes, or simply because the family shares the same eating habits and lifestyle.

In 1962 a geneticist named James Neel proposed his theory that a "thrifty gene" predisposes a person to obesity. Early humans lived as hunter-gatherers, who experienced periods of feast and famine. To adapt to extreme changes in caloric intake, they developed a gene that would allow them to store fat during the feast period, and thus prevent starvation when the food supply dwindled. If a thrifty gene does exist, it has become a liability in a society where food is plentiful all of the time.

The predisposition to put on extra weight also increases steadily as we age. Men age 65 to 74 and

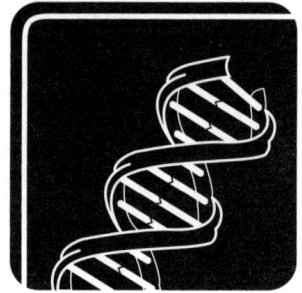

women age 55 to 64 have the highest prevalence of overweight and obesity. A decrease in physical activity is believed to be the major reason for age-related weight gain, but some studies have shown that in women, menopause can bring about a change in body composition. During menopause, lean muscle tissue may decrease, while fat increases, especially around the abdomen. Metabolism tends to slow down as people grow older, meaning that fewer calories are burned while at rest.

Some ethnic groups are hit harder by the obesity epidemic than the overall population. Blacks, Hispanics, Native Americans, and Alaska Natives gain weight at faster rates than whites, and their overall prevalence of overweight and obesity is much higher. Black women, for example, become obese at twice the rate of white women, and Hispanic men become obese (gain weight) 2.5 times faster than their Caucasian counterparts. These populations also have a higher incidence of

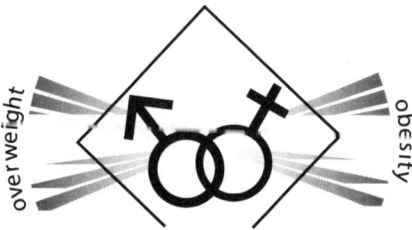

some obesity-related diseases, including diabetes, hypertension, cancer, and heart disease.

HEALTH RISKS & OBESITY

Extra weight can put your health in serious jeopardy. Obesity is associated with more than 30 medical conditions. Aside from the physical and emotional impact of these illnesses, the economic cost is staggering. The total yearly cost of obesity-related medical care is $117 billion. Following are some of the illnesses linked to obesity.

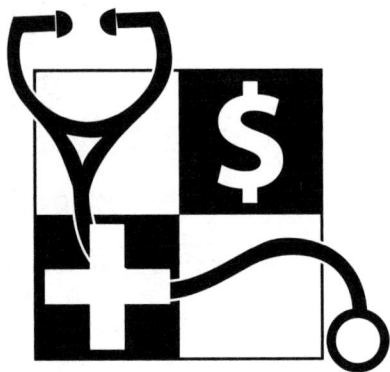

HEART DISEASE & OBESITY

Cardiovascular disease remains the number-one cause of death in the U.S., and rising obesity rates are helping to keep it there. Being overweight increases your odds of acquiring an array of risk factors for heart disease, including high LDL cholesterol and triglyceride levels, low HDL cholesterol, diabetes, and hypertension.

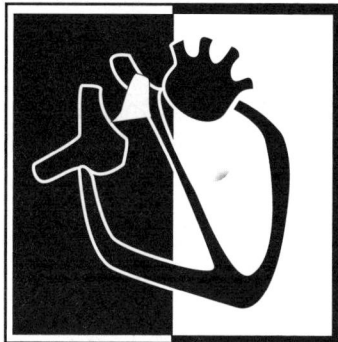

A study supported by the National Heart, Lung, and Blood Institute found that obese men have a 90% increased risk of heart failure compared to men with a healthy weight. Obesity doubles the risk of heart failure in women, according to the study, published in the *New England Journal of Medicine* in 2002. High blood pressure is also far more prevalent among people who are overweight, and the incidence rises along with weight gain.

CANCER & OBESITY

Research shows that obesity and physical inactivity may account for 25% to 30% of several major types of cancer.

An extensive American Cancer Society study on the relationship between weight and cancer risk found that the heaviest men have a 52% higher mortality rate from cancer than normal-weight men. For women, the risk is 62% higher, according to the study, published in the *New England Journal*

...obesity and physical inactivity may account for 25%-30% of several major types of cancer.

of Medicine in 2003. The results of this study added strength to previous scientific evidence linking excess weight to cancers of the uterus, kidney, esophagus, gallbladder, colon and rectum, and breast in postmenopausal women.

They also found that cancers of the liver, pancreas, prostate and stomach in men, as well as non-Hodgkin lymphoma and multiple myeloma were also affected by excess body fat.

DIABETES & OBESITY

Type 2 diabetes, formerly known as adult-onset or non-insulin-dependent diabetes, is closely linked to excess weight gain. Over 80% of people with type 2 diabetes are overweight. While this disease was once almost exclusively limited to adults, it is now frequently seen in obese children.

Approximately 800,000 new cases of diabetes are diagnosed every year. Some 90% to 95% of these cases are type 2, and nearly nine out of ten newly diagnosed type 2 diabetic patients are overweight.

In type 1 diabetes, which is typically diagnosed in children and young adults, the body stops producing insulin. There is no association between type 1 disease and weight gain. Type 2 diabetes, by contrast, usually appears in middle age or later, and while insulin is still produced, the amount is either insufficient to keep the body's glucose levels in balance, or the insulin isn't used effectively. One of the most alarming trends is the growing number of children and adolescents who are developing type 2 disease; as many as 80% of these children are overweight at the time of diagnosis.

Diabetes is a major factor in early death because it predisposes sufferers to a variety of serious complications. Diabetics are more prone to heart disease, especially atherosclerosis, and stroke. Between 10% and 21% of all people with diabetes eventually develop kidney disease or

Between 10% and 21% of all people with diabetes eventually develop kidney disease or diabetic nephropathy...

diabetic nephropathy, which is the leading cause of end-stage renal disease or renal failure. A person with renal failure must undergo dialysis or receive a kidney transplant in order to survive. Diabetes can also lead to impaired vision or even blindness as a result of diabetic retinopathy.

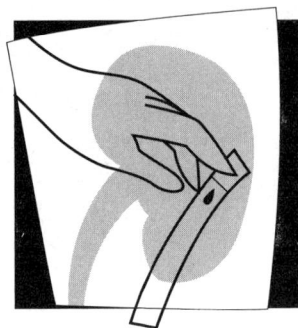

METABOLIC SYNDROME & OBESITY

Obesity is a key player in the so-called metabolic syndrome or "Syndrome X," a cluster of medical conditions that increases the risk for heart disease, stroke, and diabetes. It tends to occur in people who have excess abdominal fat. The components of metabolic syndrome include: hypertension, high triglycerides, and low blood levels of "good" HDL cholesterol. People with metabolic syndrome also tend to have insulin resistance, in which the body doesn't use insulin efficiently, and blood glucose levels are abnormally high.

Metabolic syndrome now affects 26% of all Americans. In a study published in the *New England Journal of Medicine*, researchers assessed

439 obese children for metabolic syndrome. Almost 40% of those who were moderately obese, and fully half of those with more severe obesity, had metabolic syndrome.

ARTHRITIS & OBESITY

Arthritis is one of the most common conditions in the U.S. There are several types of arthritis, but all are characterized by pain, swelling, and inflammation of the joints. Osteoarthritis, one of the most common types, is caused by a breakdown of the joint's cartilage and most often affects the joints of the knees, hips, and lower back. Obesity exacerbates the progression and severity of this disease.

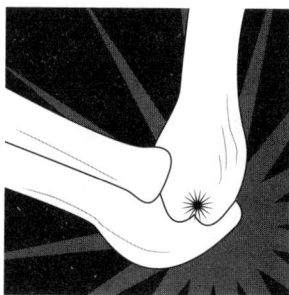

An increase in body weight puts more pressure on weight-bearing joints, which can cause the cartilage to wear away. For people with arthritis, carrying extra weight stresses the joints further. Osteoarthritis is more commonly found in women than men. And obese women have a four-fold increased risk of osteoarthritis compared to their slimmer counterparts.

SLEEP APNEA, ASTHMA, & OBESITY

Sleep apnea causes sufferers to stop breathing for short periods during sleep. Sleep apnea can be life-threatening and cause symptoms such as depression, irritability, sexual dysfunction, learning and memory difficulties, and dozing off while at work or driving. Sleep apnea boosts the risk of high blood pressure, heart attack, stroke, and congestive heart failure.

The most common form of the condition is obstructive sleep apnea, which is associated with obesity. It usually occurs when the muscles in the pharynx and tongue relax during sleep, partially blocking the airway. In obese individuals, excess fat in the neck can make the airway smaller, and thus impair breathing. Enlarged tonsils and adenoids can also exacerbate the condition.

Asthma is another breathing problem associated with obesity. Rates of both obesity and asthma have been increasing in children as well as adults, and some research has shown a strong correlation

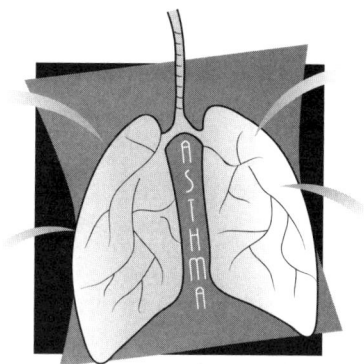

between the two. A Harvard Medical School study found that asthma is three times more likely to develop in adults who are obese. The researchers speculate that excess weight puts pressure on the airways, causing them to react more aggressively to colds and other triggers for asthma attacks. Adipose cells also synthesize cytokines, inflammatory substances that can exacerbate many pathologic processes, including chronic lung disease.

INFERTILITY & OBESITY

Excess weight has been linked to irregular menstrual cycles and the complete absence of ovulation, especially in women who are extremely obese. Polycystic ovary syndrome, a common cause of infertility in women, is a complicated hormone disorder that is associated with obesity and insulin resistance. Eventually, thyroid and adrenal gland dysfunction may occur.

Cataracts are the leading cause of blindness worldwide. They are usually considered part of the aging process, as they are quite common in older adults. But researchers at the San Francisco Department of Public Health and the Harvard School of Public Health found that as weight rises, so does the risk of cataracts. How excess weight may contribute to cataracts is not fully understood, but

Cataracts are the leading cause of blindness worldwide.

the researchers speculate that the culprit may be systemic inflammation, high blood sugar levels, or increased oxidative stress from free radicals.

DEPRESSION & OBESITY

The emotional and psychological impact of obesity is not well studied. But we do know that obesity can significantly affect a person's quality of life, mobility, and physical endurance. Obese individuals also face discrimination in the workplace, school, and in social settings.

...researchers have found an association between obesity, depression and suicidal behavior.

Several recent studies have explored the link between obesity and depression. In several studies, researchers have found an association between obesity, depression and suicidal behavior. Chronic obesity is also linked to psychiatric disorders in children and adolescents, with young boys at the greatest risk for weight-related depression. However, it is not clear whether obesity leads to depression, or vice versa. Elevated cortisol levels seem to play a significant role in both cases.

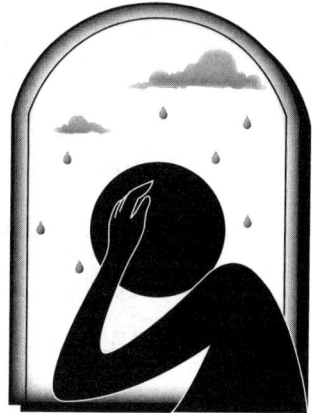

WHAT IS A HEALTHY WEIGHT?

Most of us rely on the scale to monitor our weight. But clinicians also use a tool called the body mass index (BMI), which measures weight in relation to height. The BMI closely correlates with measures of body fat, and can help predict risk of developing a health problem related to excess weight gain.

A BMI of 18.5 to 24.9 is healthy; 25 to 29.9 is overweight. A BMI of 30 or more is classified as obese. But there are limitations to the BMI. It doesn't differentiate between fat and muscle, so it can underestimate or overestimate fat in some people. Athletes, body builders, and others with a muscular build may end up having their body fat overestimated, even though they are healthy and at low risk for diabetes or heart disease. Conversely, body fat may be underestimated in an older adult or a debilitated person who has lost muscle mass.

Waist circumference is another useful measure. Research has shown that the location of body fat is often just as important as the overall BMI in assessing obesity and health risk. If fat is concentrated around your waist and abdomen (apple shape), you are more likely to develop a number of health problems than if the weight is evenly distributed—or carried primarily in the hips and thighs (pear shape). Even if your BMI is in the normal range, that spare tire increases your health risk. A waist measurement of more than 35 inches in <u>women, and 40 inches</u> in men, may put you at risk for obesity-related illnesses.

LOSING THE WEIGHT

Weight control is a life-long effort, but it is achievable. And for many, losing weight and keeping it off is well worth the effort. The end result can include better emotional and physical health, a decrease in chronic disease risk, and improved self-esteem.

Science shows that <u>the best way to lose</u> weight <u>is to alter your eating habits and increase physical activity</u>. Reducing the number of calories you take in and increasing the number you burn off is the only proven way to take off pounds. A goal of losing about a pound a week is recommended by many experts, and is relatively easy to achieve. In order to lose a pound of fat, you need to burn off or reduce dietary intake <u>by 3,500 calories</u>. So losing a pound a <u>week can be achieved by a reduction of 500 calories a day</u>. By shaving off pounds <u>slowly and steadily you are more likely to stick to a weight loss program</u>, and stay both thinner and healthier.

Ten Tips for Losing Weight & Staying Trim

1. *Exercise.* Physical activity must be part of any weight loss and maintenance program. Set a goal of 30 minutes of moderate to vigorous physical activity on most days.

2. *Eat less.* Reduce your caloric intake.

3. *Watch your portions.* In an era of supersize meals and giant portions, it is easy to overeat. When dining out, ask for a doggy bag before you begin to eat; pack half of your food to take home.

4. *Slow down.* When you eat fast, you often eat beyond your level of fullness.

5. *Address your emotions.* Don't use eating as a way to deal with stress, boredom, anger, or other negative emotions.

6. *Choose your calories carefully.* Eat plenty of fruits and vegetables, which are high in nutrition and low in calories and fat.

7. *Fat-free is not calorie free.* A product labeled fat-free may be packed with calories.

8. *Watch liquid calories.* Many calories lurk in everyday drinks. A Starbucks caffè mocha with whipped cream is worth 260 calories and 12 grams of fat using non-fat milk.

9. *Control snacking.* Keep healthier snacks on hand so you'll be less likely to load up on sugary foods with no nutritive value. Fresh fruit, low-fat yogurt, hard-boiled eggs, baby carrots and celery sticks, or low-fat whole grain crackers are some healthier alternatives.

10. *Hold on to your new weight.* Maintaining a healthy weight means changing your lifestyle, not trying out a one-shot diet. Keep up good eating habits, keep exercising, and continue working on the emotional triggers that tempt you to overeat.

As well as diet and exercise, pharmaceuticals have been used successfully for losing weight, and are especially helpful for those who are very obese. Bontril, Desoxyn, Ionamin, and Adipex-P, which were approved by the FDA years ago, suppress the appetite and increase the metabolic rate. These drugs are only effective in the short term, as your body soon begins to build up tolerance to them. And, of course, there are side effects such as elevated heart rate.

Weight loss drugs have been a disappointment. Meridia, approved in 1997, suppressed the appetite but was removed from the market. Xenical, approved in 1999, interferes with fat absorption in the intestines. Another once promising drug in clinical trials, Accomplia, reduced food cravings but has also been placed on hold. So far, complications have limited clinical usefulness. Some newer drugs are discussed in **Chapter 7**.

Surgery is an option for people who cannot be helped by more conservative approaches.

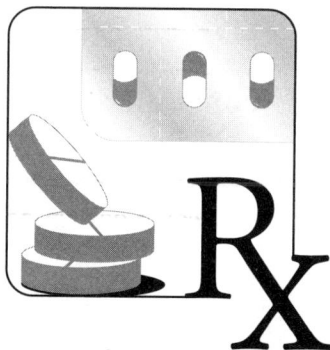

It may be a suitable choice for those who are extremely obese, especially if they have a serious obesity-related medical condition.

OBESITY: A PUBLIC HEALTH PROBLEM

Tackling obesity at a national level is a monumental task. However, researchers and government officials have launched a number of efforts aimed at reducing obesity in the U.S. The U.S. Department of Health and Human Services has begun the Healthy Lifestyles & Disease Prevention initiative, which includes multimedia public service advertisements about exercise and diet, and an interactive website that instructs people on how to reach their weight loss goal.

An FDA initiative with the motto, "calories count" is aimed at reducing obesity rates in the U.S. It focuses on improving food labeling, encouraging restaurants to provide nutritional information to consumers, and revising its own guidelines for developing drugs to treat obesity.

Yet organizations such as the Center for Science in the Public Interest, along with a number of scientists and physicians, believe that more aggressive action needs to be taken.

Their proposals include: restricting television advertising of high-calorie, low-nutrient foods to children; requiring fast food and other chain restaurants to provide information about calorie content on menus; and lowering prices of fruits and vegetables. They also recommend subsidizing the cost of nutritious, low-calorie foods by raising the price of high-calorie, low-nutrient foods in vending machines and school cafeterias. Perhaps we could return to the concept of parents as role models.

IMPROVE HEALTH BY DROPPING THE POUNDS

Taking off excess weight can reverse a number of obesity-related illnesses—and reduce the severity of symptoms. Research has found that weight loss reduces triglycerides, total cholesterol, and LDL cholesterol levels, and raises HDL cholesterol. Blood pressure also drops. In people with type 2 diabetes, weight loss improves glucose control. In some people, blood sugar returns to normal with weight loss. Sleep apnea symptoms become less severe or resolve completely, menstrual cycles become more regular, and symptoms of osteoarthritis improve. Overall, weight loss leads to a better quality of life.

Canadian researchers found that weight loss improved lung function in obese women with asthma, according to a study published in the journal *Chest* in June 2004.

Scientists in Sweden noted that the long-term effects of weight loss not only improved overall health, but also reduced the use of medications needed to treat cardiovascular disease and diabetes. Long-term weight loss also decreases the overall costs of treating diabetes and heart disease.

THE BOTTOM LINE

Reducing overweight and obesity unquestionably improves our physical and emotional health. It also relieves our healthcare system of the need to spend billions of dollars to care for those with obesity-related diseases.

In the following chapters, we'll show you how to achieve your weight loss goals, and improve your health. We'll discuss the pros and cons of various

Reducing overweight and obesity

Improving physical and emotional health

weight loss strategies, ranging from popular diets to bariatric surgery to cutting-edge medications. After reading this book, you may just find you have the tools to achieve a "weight perfect" lifestyle.

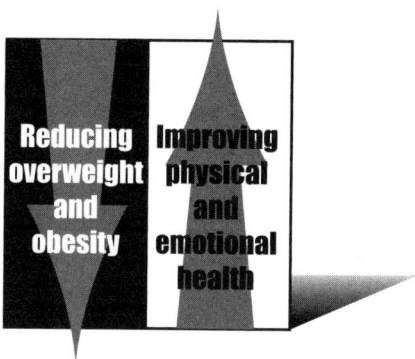

EIGHT WEIGHT LOSS MYTHS

#1: Certain foods can burn fat and speed weight loss.

No foods can burn fat—even very low-calorie foods such as grapefruit, celery, and cabbage soup. Foods containing caffeine may speed up the body's metabolism for a short time. Over the long-term, however, drinking beverages with caffeine will probably not have much effect on weight loss. Calorie content itself is the only component of food that has an effect on weight loss or gain.

#2: Skipping meals is an effective way to lose weight.

Studies show that people who skip breakfast and eat fewer times during the day tend to be heavier than people who eat a healthy breakfast and eat four or five times a day. Skipping meals may lead

Body Mass Index (BMI)

A measure of body weight relative to height. BMI can be used to determine if people are at a healthy weight, overweight, or obese. To figure out BMI, use the following formula:

BMI = weight (lbs) x 703 ÷ height (inches) x height (inches)

A body mass index (BMI) of 18.5 up to 24.9 refers to a healthy weight, a BMI of 25 up to 29.9 refers to overweight and a BMI of 30 or higher refers to obese.

Classification of Overweight & Obesity by BMI, Waist Circumference, & Associated Disease Risks

	BMI (kg/m^2)	Obesity Class	Disease Risk* Relative to Normal Weight & Waist Circumference	
			Men 102 cm (40") or less Women 88 cm (35") or less	Men > 102 cm (40") Women > 88 cm (35")
Underweight	< 18.5		–	–
Normal	18.5 - 24.9		–	–
Overweight	25.0 - 29.9		Increased	High
Obesity	30.0 - 34.9	I	High	Very High
Obesity	35.0 - 39.9	II	Very High	Very High
Extreme Obesity	40.0 +	III	Extremely High	Extremely High

* Disease risk for type 2 diabetes, hypertension, and CVD.
+ Increased waist circumference can also be a marker for increased risk even in persons of normal weight.

Source: National Institutes of Health. Available at: *www.nhlbi.nih.gov/health/public/ heart/obesity/lose_wt/bmi_dis.htm*. Accessed July 2018.

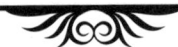

to feeling hungrier later on in the day, and may result in overeating or even bingeing. Eating smaller meals spaced throughout the day also helps control appetite. So eating frequent, small meals consisting of healthy, low-fat/calorie foods may help you lose weight.

#3: Eating after 8 p.m. causes weight gain.

The timing of your meals has minimal impact on weight gain. The amount and kind of foods you eat, as well as your physical activity, are the only things that determine whether you lose, maintain or gain weight. If you'd like to snack before going to bed, consider the number of calories you've already consumed that day.

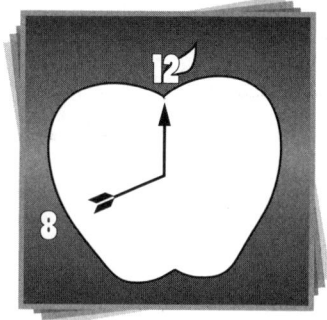

#4: Lifting weights is not beneficial to weight loss because it causes too much "bulking up."

Lifting weights or other muscle strengthening exercises may actually help maintain body weight or speed weight loss. These exercises build muscles, which burn off more calories than fat. With more muscle, you'll burn more calories—even when sitting still. Only intense strength training combined with a certain genetic background will produce large, bulky muscles.

#5: Nuts are fattening and should be avoided when trying to lose weight.

Although relatively high in calories, nuts can be part of a healthy weight loss program. They are a good source of protein, dietary fiber, minerals, and

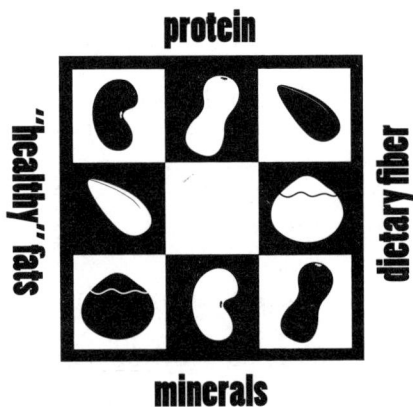

unsaturated ("healthy") fats. For those attempting to lose weight, controlling portion size is beneficial. One-third cup of nuts has about 270 calories.

#6: Eating red meat is unhealthy and makes losing weight harder.

Eating lean cuts and small amounts of red meat can be part of a healthy weight loss plan. Red meat, chicken, pork and fish contain some cholesterol and saturated fat, but also have nutrients such as protein, iron, and zinc. Trimming visible fat before cooking meat and controlling portion size can help in your weight loss efforts. A serving of meat is about 3 to 4 ounces of cooked meat, the size of a deck of cards.

#7: Dairy products are fattening and unhealthy.

Dairy products are rich in important nutrients such as protein, calcium, and vitamin D. Reduced and nonfat dairy products are readily available, however, and are just as nutritious as whole milk yogurt, milk and cheese. If you are lactose intolerant or choose not to use animal products, try eating fortified foods or dark leafy greens to obtain calcium and vitamin D.

#8: Switching to a vegetarian diet leads to losing weight and being healthier.

A vegetarian diet does not necessarily entail eating more nutritious and/or lower calorie foods. Research shows, however, that people who follow a vegetarian diet eat fewer calories and less fat than non-vegetarians, and tend to have lower body weights relative to their heights.

If you are a vegetarian, choosing low-fat foods may help you lose weight. When trying to lose or keep off pounds, it's also important to limit high-calorie foods and those with little or no nutritional value.

Some crucial nutrients commonly found in non-vegetarian eating plans—such as iron, vitamin D, vitamin B_{12}, zinc and calcium—can be difficult to incorporate into a vegetarian diet. So if you do choose a vegetarian diet, make sure you are getting all essential nutrients in your meals.

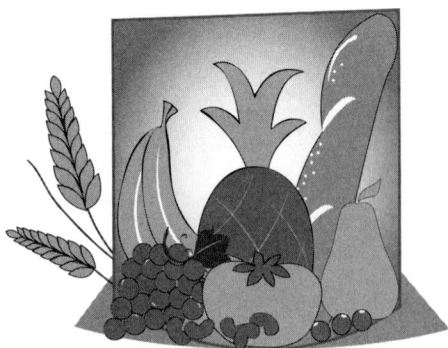

The Doctor's Dilemma: Tackling Obesity in 15 Minutes

The Scenario: An obese 46-year-old woman asks her doctor to help her lose weight, saying she just can't stay on a diet. But it's a busy day, and her doctor has only 15 minutes to give her. Still the physician knows that a curt, "eat less, exercise more" answer would be ineffective.

Yet, even when physicians are pressed for time, it is possible to start patients on an effective weight loss program—even in just 15 minutes.

The best bet is to assess a patient properly—including her weight and health risks, current lifestyle, and previous weight loss attempts. Then fashion a plan to suit the individual.

Suggest a diet and type of exercise that the patient thinks would be enjoyable and sustainable. Recommend a few lifestyle changes the patient can make easily—cutting down on portion sizes, bringing a lunch to work instead of eating out, or increasing vegetable intake. And finally, consider using medication if the patient's condition warrants it.

It's also helpful to suggest resources that the patient can use to stay on target in their weight loss efforts, such as publications, books, support groups, commercial or non-profit weight loss plans, and consultation with a dietitian.

Source: Hensrud DD. Tackling obesity in a 15-minute office visit: physicians can start patients on an effective weight-loss program, despite time constrains. *Postgrad Med.* 2004 Jan; 115(1):59-61.

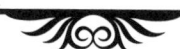

Chapter 2

the food-sleep connection: insomnia & obesity

"A good laugh and a long sleep are the best cures in the doctor's book."

~ *Irish Proverb*

"No day is so bad it can't be fixed with a nap."

~ *Carrie Snow, comedian*

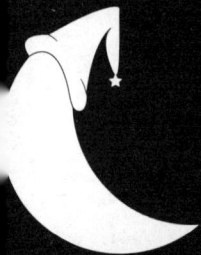

We've all experienced the head-nodding effects of sleep deprivation at one time or another. During class or a long afternoon at work, even driving a car, our concentration ebbs, our eyelids become heavy, and we must fight to stay awake. At the very least, sleep deprivation symptoms are an annoyance. In the case of driving or performing other critical tasks, sleep deprivation is dangerous. But there is a relationship between sleep deprivation and obesity. In fact, recent studies point to definitive links between chronic lack of sleep and weight gain.

Sleep deprivation can be the result of lifestyle choices or medical conditions such as depression, anxiety, menopause, pregnancy, and pain syndromes. It can also result from shift work, frequent travel across time zones, medication side effects, clinical sleep disorders, and caregiving responsibilities.

In response to ever-busier lifestyles, Americans are cutting back on sleep. The average amount of sleep for a U.S. citizen in 1910 was nine hours. By 1997, it had dropped to seven hours. In their 2002 Sleep in America Poll, the National Sleep Foundation found that respondents slept about 6.9 hours during the week on average, and 7.5 hours on the weekends. On weeknights, 15% reported sleeping less than six hours and 39% said they slept less than seven hours. Clearly, those statistics have deteriorated in recent years.

Sleep-related problems affect between 50 million and 70 million Americans of all ages, according to the National Center on Sleep Disorders Research. Approximately 30% to 40% of the adult population is affected by insomnia, the most common type of sleep disorder. Insomnia is defined as having difficulty falling asleep, difficulty staying asleep, or fragmented sleep.

Interestingly, the increasing prevalence of sleep deprivation in the U.S. over the past 35 years has occurred in tandem with the rising rates of obesity. In fact, several studies have suggested that two epidemics—obesity and sleeplessness—are linked. Although the exact relationship is still unclear, a number of hypotheses have emerged.

In a groundbreaking 1999 study, published in the British medical journal *The Lancet*, researchers from the University of Chicago found that chronic sleep loss can reduce the capacity of the body to process and store carbohydrates. Lack of sleep may also interfere with the secretion of key hormones that influence weight gain.

The relationship between body fat and sleep duration was examined in a study of almost 7,000 German children, published in the *International Journal of Obesity & Related Metabolic Disorders*. The researchers found that the prevalence of obesity decreased as the amount of sleeping time increased. This relationship appeared to be independent of other risk factors for childhood obesity.

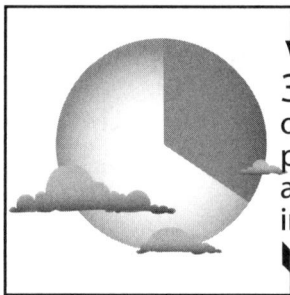

30%–40% of the adult population is affected by insomnia.

The Impact of Insomnia

- People with insomnia are four times as likely to suffer from depression as people who sleep well.

- Lack of sleep may contribute to illnesses such as heart disease

- People with insomnia may miss more time from work, or receive fewer promotions.

- After a poor night's sleep, many people report accomplishing fewer daily tasks and enjoying activities less.

Source: National Sleep Foundation

Swiss and American researchers discovered much the same thing when they studied a group of 500 adults over a 13-year period. In the June 2004 issue of *Sleep*, they reported that as sleep time decreased, the BMI (body mass index) increased.

HORMONES: THE KEY TO IT ALL

During normal sleep, the brain moves through a succession of five recurring stages. Sleep disorders that affect the quality, duration, and onset of sleep may disrupt endocrine functions.

A number of these hormones are linked to weight gain, including growth hormone (GH),

How Sleep Deprivation Leads to Weight Gain

- Growth hormone levels decrease
- Thyroid function is compromised
- Insulin sensitivity is compromised
- Leptin levels decrease (appetite increases)
- Ghrelin levels increase (appetite increases)
- Cortisol levels increase (stress eating increases)

Leptin is a hormone synthesized by adipose cells. It signals the appetite center in the hypothalamus to stop eating when normal weight is exceeded.

Ghrelin is a hormone released by gastric cells when the stomach is empty. It signals the hypothalamus to increase food intake. Ghrelin levels are sharply reduced after gastric bypass surgery.

thyroid hormones, insulin and cortisol—the "stress hormone." Other hormones that affect weight gain include melatonin, testosterone, estrogen, leptin, and ghrelin.

GROWTH HORMONE: THE DOMINO EFFECT

Sleep deprivation—especially lack of deep sleep (stage 4) and REM (dream stage) sleep—interferes with the production of growth hormone (GH). GH is important because it helps us maintain a healthy weight and muscle mass, and influences metabolism. Decreasing production of GH has a domino effect. Levels of other hormones that influence metabolism and weight then change, and the result is often weight gain.

The suppression of growth hormone, which occurs during the normal aging process or from a chronic lack of sleep, appears to have a significant effect on both body weight and composition. Decreasing levels of GH are associated with aging fat gain and decreased muscle mass.

Growth hormone has a significant effect on our ability to metabolize proteins, lipids, and carbohydrates. It also stimulates adipocytes (fat cells) to break down triglycerides.

GH also affects us indirectly—through its role in stimulating the liver and other tissues to secrete a hormone called insulin-like growth factor-1 (IGF-1). Nearly every cell in our body is affected by IGF-1, which is essential to normal growth and plays a key role in muscle and nerve development.

A number of studies have shown correlations between low GH levels and obesity. Generally, people who are obese have lower levels of GH than normal-weight people. While the exact mechanism behind this phenomenon remains unclear, Italian researchers found that low GH levels in obese people can be normalized by weight reduction. Reporting in the *International Journal of Obesity and Related Metabolic Disorders*, the researchers found that normal secretion of GH began spontaneously when weight loss occurred. Treatment with GH supplementation also resulted in improved metabolism and body composition.

In a study from St. Louis University, obese people who were treated with GH experienced normalized levels of IGF-1. As a result, they lost weight from fat and not muscle, and improved their cholesterol levels.

Fortunately, we can stimulate GH production by increasing our physical activity. In their book *Protein Power*, Drs. Mary Dan and Michael Eades report that resistance training (weight lifting) is the best form of exercise for stimulating the release of GH. Increased muscle mass sets our body's metabolic rate higher so that it burns more calories at rest. A higher metabolic rate enables us to burn more calories even while we're simply sitting at a computer or watching television. Curiously, alcohol can suppress GH production.

CORTISOL & SLEEP

Cortisol is commonly known as the "stress hormone" because it's secreted in response to a stressed or agitated state. Any type of physical or mental stress can increase the production and release of cortisol, including illness, surgery, extreme temperatures, or psychological problems. However, cortisol is far more than just a marker of stress levels. A steroid hormone produced in our adrenal glands, cortisol is necessary for blood pressure regulation, cardiovascular function, and carbohydrate and protein metabolism.

Chronically elevated cortisol levels result in muscle loss, increase in body fat, immune suppression, and reduced ability to repair tissue damage. Research has shown that cortisol levels tend to be elevated in people suffering from

Exercise & Sleep

- Consistent exercise improves the quality of sleep by re-oxygenating the body, improving circulation, and normalizing circadian rhythms.

- Avoid exercising during the 3 hours before bedtime, because exercise is stimulating and can increase core temperature, reducing melatonin synthesis.

- Strenuous exercise close to bedtime can raise cortisol levels, make your muscles sore, and keep you tossing and turning.

- Relaxing exercise like yoga or Pilates stretches and relaxes muscles and helps induce sleep.

sleep deprivation and depression. In one study, a research team at the Sleep Research and Treatment Center of the Pennsylvania State University College of Medicine found that cortisol levels were significantly higher in a group of chronic insomniacs over a 24-hour period. The results of their study, which was published in the *Journal of Clinical Endocrinology & Metabolism*, also showed that the insomniacs with the worst sleep disturbances secreted the highest amounts of cortisol.

Chronic high levels of cortisol may also increase our appetite and cravings for certain foods, especially carbohydrates and sweets. As a result, when we're sleep-deprived, we may feel hungry even though we're eating adequate amounts of food.

SLEEP APNEA: A LINK TO LOW THYROID LEVELS?

Decreased levels of thyroid hormones, or hypothyroidism, can lower basal metabolic rate. So, as metabolism slows down, weight gain results. In addition, people who have hypothyroidism are chronically tired—often too tired to exercise—making it more difficult for them to burn calories and lose weight.

Hypothyroidism has been associated with sleep apnea.

Obstructive sleep apnea, in which obstruction in the pharynx blocks air flow to the lungs, is associated with obesity and hypothyroidism. The airway can be blocked by the tongue, tonsils, or uvula, or even relaxed throat muscles. Sometimes the structure of the jaw and airway can be a factor in sleep apnea, as can obstruction of the nasal passages. In obese people, excess fatty tissue in the neck and throat can make the airway smaller, and thus impair breathing. While not everyone with obstructive sleep apnea is overweight, it has been identified as a major risk factor.

People with obstructive sleep apnea stop breathing for short periods of time during the night because of airway blockage. The pauses in breathing are short, generally no longer than 10 or 20 seconds. In mild cases, these pauses may occur only a few times during the night, but those with severe apnea can experience significantly more. Fortunately, the majority of people wake up during an episode of sleep apnea. As soon as they are awakened, muscle activity in the tongue and throat increases, and the airway enlarges. Breathing begins again, and the person usually falls back to sleep immediately. This cycle repeats itself many times during the night.

Although most people have no memory of them, these nocturnal pauses and awakenings do interrupt sleep and can lead to daytime sleepiness, poor concentration, and performance problems. Sleep apnea can be life-threatening and cause symptoms such as depression, irritability, sexual dysfunction, learning and memory difficulties, and dozing off while at work or driving. Sleep apnea can increase

Sleep apnea can increase the risk of high blood pressure, heart attack and stroke.

the risk of high blood pressure, heart attack, stroke, congestive heart failure, and arrhythmias.

Sleep apnea is diagnosed with a polysomnogram, which monitors brain waves, muscle tension, eye movement, respiration, and oxygen levels in the blood. It also involves audio monitoring of sounds such as snoring and gasping—both common in sleep apnea. The test is noninvasive and is performed overnight, either in a sleep lab or in your own home.

The most common treatment for sleep apnea is continuous positive airway pressure (CPAP), which involves wearing a face mask while sleeping. The mask is connected to a machine that forces air through the nasal passages. The air pressure is adjusted so that it keeps the throat open during sleep, thus preventing apneic episodes. In some patients, a dental appliance known as a mandibular advancement device helps improve position of the lower jaw, facilitating air flow. Surgery is sometimes performed to remove tonsils and adenoids that may be blocking the airway, or to remove excess tissue at the back of the throat.

Losing weight is frequently helpful in treating sleep apnea. Even a 10% weight loss can decrease the number of sleep apnea events during the night. And for patients with hypothyroidism, thyroid replacement therapy may successfully treat sleep apnea, as well as help in weight loss. Therapy with growth hormone has also been shown to be helpful.

SLEEP PROBLEMS AT MIDLIFE

Testosterone fires both the male and female sex drive and helps burn fat. It is also a strong GH stimulant. Around midlife, testosterone and GH levels may drop in men, while relative estrogen levels increase. Sleep can be disturbed from stress, snoring, and other factors. The result is that men gain weight, grow paunchy with increased breast tissue, and have a significantly lowered libido.

In menopausal women, estrogen levels drop—resulting in decreased sex drive, hot flashes and weight gain. Hot flashes can disrupt the quality of a woman's sleep, and may cause frequent awakenings during the night. If a woman's hot flashes are severe, she can take hormone replacement therapy (HRT). Even low doses for 2 to 3 years may help.

Hot flashes can disrupt the quality of a woman's sleep...

Women who do not experience hot flashes can also suffer from insomnia during menopause, however. Prescription sleep medications can help.

Testosterone may improve the quality of sleep and secretion of GH in both men and women, according to some experts. Small doses of testosterone may give women more energy, a higher libido, and help them to lose body fat during menopause. Several studies have shown that when testosterone levels are increased in either men or women, sleep and general well being improves, GH levels increase, and body fat decreases.

Testosterone supplementation, however, is controversial. Some researchers are concerned that testosterone supplements may increase the risk of prostate cancer and accelerate coronary artery disease in men. It can also cause increased body hair and acne in women.

SEROTONIN: BETTER SLEEP, BETTER MOOD

Serotonin is a neurotransmitter that is produced after eating carbohydrates. Serotonin induces relaxation and promotes sleep, especially stage 4 sleep, which is crucial to secreting growth hormone. GH helps burn stored fat and maintains normal muscle mass and weight.

Low serotonin levels signal a need for carbohydrates, and we begin to crave these foods. As a result of eating carbohydrates, tryptophan levels increase and enhance release of serotonin. After dining on carbohydrates, serotonin levels increase, and we often feel more relaxed—even sleepy.

Can carbohydrates increase the ability to sleep, and thus cut down on weight gain? Carbohydrates must be eaten with little-to-no protein in order to produce serotonin, and aid sleep, says Judith Wurtman, an MIT researcher and nutritionist. Dr. Wurtman explains that some people are "carbohydrate cravers" who need to eat a certain amount of carbohydrates a day to keep their mood on an even keel. These people generally experience carbohydrate cravings in the late afternoon or early evening. Eating a food that's sweet or starchy can often help them relax and get a good night's sleep.

Many researchers agree that early evening is the best time of day to eat carbohydrates to ensure relaxation and to attain deep sleep.

OUR SLEEP-WAKE CYCLE: HOW IT AFFECTS WEIGHT GAIN

Most of us have experienced "jet lag" when we travel to a different time zone. This is caused by a disruption in our circadian rhythm, or our sleep-wake cycle.

Circadian rhythm is controlled by the hypothalamus and pineal gland. Our brain relies on environmental time cues such as sunlight, food, noise, or social interaction to set our internal "clock" or sleep-wake cycle. The active secretion of melatonin, a hormone produced by the pineal

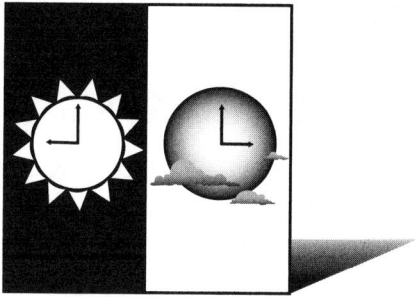

gland, plays a large part in setting our internal clock, and enables us to get a good night's rest. Melatonin secretion begins each day at sunset. As this hormone is released into the bloodstream, we may begin to feel sleepy or less alert. Melatonin levels remain elevated in the blood for about 12 hours, and begin to decrease as the daylight hours draw near. Our daytime levels of melatonin are normally extremely low.

Shift workers, people who work the late night or "graveyard" shift, also experience disruption of their circadian rhythm. They must slumber during the day, when melatonin secretion is decreased and "cues" such as sunlight and noise signal them to stay awake, so their sleep quality is often poor. When beginning late night shift work, people often experience a substantial loss of sleep, particularly stage 4 or delta wave sleep, needed to make GH, reduce cortisol levels, and burn fat. So it's understandable that those who work from late afternoon into the early hours of the morning tend to have problems with obesity.

Disrupted circadian rhythm usually results in changes in production of growth hormone, thyroid hormone, and insulin, all of which affect weight. It can also engender cravings for sugars and starches because of decreased serotonin levels.

Increased appetite and craving for carbohydrate-rich foods are pronounced in people with seasonal affective disorder (SAD), a type of depression related to seasonal changes in daylight and darkness. People with SAD typically experience disruptions in circadian rhythm.

The onset of SAD is in late autumn; it peaks in winter, then subsides with the return of spring. It may be related to increases in blood melatonin levels, which result from the longer periods of darkness, as well as lower levels of serotonin. People with SAD often have chronically elevated insulin levels as well, which may also put them at greater risk for obesity.

SAD can also affect those who live or work in badly lit environments, even in the summer months. People who have SAD often feel lethargic

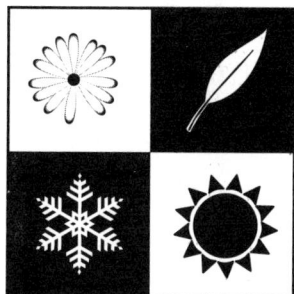

The onset of SAD is in late autumn; it peaks in winter, then subsides with the return of spring.

and lack energy. This decrease in activity further slows their metabolism, which also contributes to weight gain.

SAD patients can be treated with light therapy to counteract high melatonin levels. However, they also need to eat balanced carbohydrate and protein diets in order to raise their serotonin levels and decrease body weight.

A moderate amount of aerobic exercise decreases melatonin levels and helps to produce endorphins. Exercise should preferably be done outdoors in available daylight, or in a room lit by a full spectrum light or an Ott lamp. Regular aerobic exercise also speeds up metabolism and helps limit weight gain.

When deprived of sleep, many of us tend to eat more than is necessary. Some research suggests that fatigue produces a craving for sweets and other foods high in carbohydrates.

When our blood sugar levels drop, our body signals us to reach for something starchy or sweet to eat. If we follow these cues and have a meal, our blood sugar level rises and we feel better. However, the fatigue that comes with sleep deprivation often feels similar to the tiredness produced by real hunger. So instead of taking a nap or going to bed earlier—in order to address our fatigue—we eat to feel more energetic.

There are some nutrition rules that most sleep experts agree can help you sleep. Try out these tips to get a good night's rest.

- Avoid stimulating foods like chocolate, alcohol, caffeine-containing drinks, MSG, and tobacco.
- Eat foods high in tryptophan a few hours before bedtime; some good choices include turkey, bananas, figs, dates, yogurt, milk, tuna, whole grain crackers, and nut butter. Or try healthy

complex carbohydrates such as whole wheat pasta, oatmeal, or cream of wheat with milk.

~ Avoid heavy or spicy foods just prior to bedtime. These meals can interfere with sleep by causing heartburn.

~ Limit liquids of any kind for at least 90 minutes before bedtime, if the need to urinate awakens you during the night.

DETECTING SLEEP ABNORMALITIES

If you are experiencing sleep problems, it's important to determine the cause. Testing can rule out medical conditions such as sleep apnea, adrenal tumors, hyperthyroidism, or underlying psychological or neurologic problems like Alzheimer's disease. Depression and anxiety disorders can significantly impact sleep patterns.

Depression and anxiety disorders can significantly impact sleep patterns.

Sleep clinics use a number of tests to determine the cause of sleep problems. They include:

Polysomnogram. This painless, overnight test examines sleep cycles and stages by monitoring brain waves, electrical activity of muscles, eye movement, breathing rate, blood pressure, blood oxygen saturation, and heart rhythm. Electrodes are placed on the face, scalp, chest, abdomen, and legs. A small probe is placed on the index finger to record blood oxygen levels. Polysomnograms are very useful for diagnosing a number of sleep disorders, including insomnia, sleep apnea, and nocturnal seizures.

Multiple Sleep Latency Test. This test monitors sleep patterns, and can be helpful in diagnosing sleep disorders. Electrodes placed on the face and head record eye movement, muscle tone, and brain waves during sleep. The MSLT is done during the daytime, usually following a polysomnogram. Sleep patterns are studied during a series of four or five 30-minute naps at two-hour intervals.

PRESCRIPTION SLEEP AIDS: WHICH ONES ARE BEST?

Prescription medications that aid sleep are called hypnotics. These include benzodiazepines, such as *triazolam* (Halcion) and non-benzodiazepines such as *zolpidem* (Ambien). Use of high doses

What About OTC Sleep Aids?

- *Over-the-counter sleep aids* include antihistamines such as Nytol, Sominex, and Unisom. These OTC sleep aids should only be used for a short period of time. The most common side effects of OTC sleep aids are constipation, dry mouth, and difficulty urinating. Ironically, they can also cause nervousness and insomnia, rather than drowsiness. These drugs are anticholinergic and also cause confusion, tachycardia and ataxia. They should not be used in people over age 60.

- *Herbal supplements:* Chamomile, valerian root, hops, lavender, catnip, and passionflower are among the herbs used to produce sleep. They can be purchased as capsules, as a liquid tincture, or as a tea. Herbal remedies are generally considered safe, but as they have not undergone stringent testing, and their benefits are not scientifically proven. Never combine herbal products with prescription medications.

- *Melatonin:* Normally secreted by the pineal gland, this hormone signals the body that it is time for sleep. It is available as a supplement, and is most commonly used for sleep disturbances related to jet lag, insomnia, and shift work. Research on melatonin's efficacy is inconclusive, although some studies have found it to be useful in alleviating jet lag. Side effects at the recommended dosages (.3 to 3 mg) are uncommon, but melatonin has been known to cause itching, abnormal heartbeats, and headaches. It should not be used by pregnant or nursing women or by individuals with allergies or autoimmune disorders.

- *Mineral supplements:* Calcium and magnesium are essential minerals and perform many functions in the body. They can also help induce restful sleep, as they relax the central nervous system and muscles. A supplement taken at night with food may help you sleep. Patients with kidney stones should not take calcium supplements.

of hypnotics with longer half-lives (they remain effective in the body for a longer period of time) can increase the risk of rebound insomnia and other side effects. Rebound insomnia occurs when someone stops taking the medication, and then suffers insomnia that is worse than what they experienced before treatment.

Studies show hypnotics can shorten the time it takes to fall asleep and increase sleep time. Hypnotics also decrease night and early morning awakenings and may improve sleep quality. Research indicates that some hypnotics, particularly non-benzodiazepines such as *zolpidem* (Ambien), *zaleplon* (Sonata), and *eszopiclone* (Lunesta) provide better quality sleep than benzodiazepines—older drugs for treatment of insomnia. Unlike benzodiazepines, drugs such as *zolpidem* and *zaleplon* do not disrupt normal sleep architecture. Because they have a short half-life (remaining in the body for only a few hours) they are not generally addictive, and also carry less risk of side effects such as daytime sleepiness, rebound insomnia, and memory impairment.

Prescription Sleep Medications

- **Ambien** *(Zolpidem)* – nonbenzodiazepine; half-life of 2.5 hours; available as a tablet, extended release, oral spray, and sub-lingual

- **Sonata** *(Zaleplon)* – nonbenzodiazepine; half-life of 1 hour; may help with middle-of-the-night awakening

- **Lunesta** *(Eszopiclone)* – nonbenzodiazepine; half-life of 6 hours; may help with sleep maintenance

- **Rozerem** *(Ramelteon)* – a melatonin receptor agonist; half-life of 1–5 hours; can be used in patients with mild to moderate sleep apnea or COPD

- **Belsomra** *(Suvorexant)* – an orexin-receptor antagonist which blocks wakefulness signals; may cause next day somnolence; expensive

- *Doxepin, ultra low dose* – tricyclic antidepressant; half-life of 15 hours; used for sleep maintenance insomnia

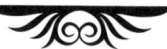

Sleep medications should never be combined with alcohol or drugs for anxiety.

There are certain risks to taking hypnotics. Some hypnotics, particularly those with a longer half-life, may cause daytime drowsiness. In fact, people who take long-acting sleep medications are at increased risk for car accidents. The sedating effects of these medicines also increases the risk for falls, especially in the elderly. In people who have sleep apnea or other respiratory conditions, hypnotics can impair breathing. Those with a shorter half-life are less likely to cause respiratory problems.

THE BOTTOM LINE

Fortunately, most sleep disorders can be treated with lifestyle changes and/or prescription medication. Patients often need to allocate more time for sleep over the course of a busy week, and efforts to reduce tension and stress are often helpful. Exercise also improves sleep quality. It might also help to seek the advice and help of a medical professional to treat an underlying condition such as depression, anxiety, chronic pain, or thyroid problems.

The truth is that it is difficult to maintain a healthy weight, lose weight, or keep lost pounds from returning if you are not getting the sleep that your body needs. Adequate and restful sleep is one of the essential components of successful weight loss and maintenance.

Quick Tips: Good Sleep Habits

To improve the duration and quality of your sleep, try these tips:

- Keep a regular sleep schedule by going to bed and waking up at the same time every day. Don't try to make up for lost sleep on weekends.

- Create a restful place to sleep. Adjust your bedroom's temperature so it's comfortable for you. The optimum temperature for sleep is between 65–67° F. Consider a new mattress, pillows, window shades or an eye mask.

- Try not to take naps; they can decrease your ability to sleep at night by reducing sleep urgency.

- If you can't get to sleep, don't just lie in bed. Get up and do something you find restful—reading or meditating works for many people.

- Avoid caffeine after 2 p.m.

- Avoid alcohol within 3–4 hours of bedtime—as alcohol is metabolized by the liver, sleep disruption can occur.

- Don't go to bed hungry, but avoid large, heavy meals or spicy foods within three hours of bedtime to reduce the risk of GERD.

- Resist the temptation to use electronic devices within one hour of bedtime.

- Stop work-related activities, problem-solving, or serious discussions within two hours of bedtime.

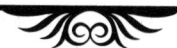

Chapter 3

medical conditions & weight gain

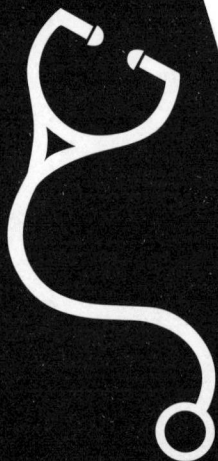

"The greatest wealth is health."

～ *Virgil*

We all know that if we don't follow a healthy diet and exercise regularly, we're likely to gain weight. There is also growing evidence that genetics plays a part in weight gain. But sometimes—often unknowingly—people put on extra pounds because of a medical condition or the medications they take.

Certain medical conditions and medications not only cause weight gain, but impede a person's ability to lose weight. These illnesses include polycystic ovary syndrome, thyroid disease and Cushing's Syndrome. Disorders such as multiple sclerosis, Parkinson's disease, and fibromyalgia can also lead to weight gain, often because fatigue makes it difficult to exercise. And a variety of medications, including widely-used antidepressants and diabetes drugs, can increase appetite or the tendency to gain weight.

Even if you take a medication or have a condition that causes you to put on extra pounds, it is possible to control your weight. And weight loss may have a hidden benefit: It may help alleviate symptoms in some chronic illnesses.

The most common type of thyroid disease, hypothyroidism, is a potentially serious problem—affecting one in six people, according to the Colorado Thyroid Disease Prevalence Study.

One of the symptoms of hypothyroidism is weight gain. Other symptoms include fatigue, sensitivity to cold, poor memory, constipation, slow heartbeat, and thick puffy dry skin.

If left untreated, hypothyroidism can lead to complications such as elevated cholesterol levels, heart disease, swelling of the face or around the eyes, infertility, muscle weakness, irregular periods, and osteoporosis. Because hypothyroidism decreases metabolism, weight gain is a very common symptom.

A TSH (blood test) is the most sensitive way to diagnose thyroid disease, and treatment of hypothyroidism is quite straightforward. The most common treatment is a once daily dose of the synthetic thyroid drug *levothyroxine* (brand names such as Synthroid, Levothroid, Levosine or Levo-T).

In the setting of hypothyroidism, exercise can increase fitness and energy levels, reduce depression, and lower stress levels—not to mention helping to control weight. Weight training can rebuild muscle lost because of thyroid imbalance.

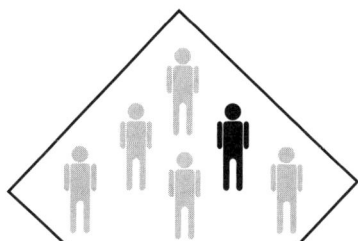
Hypothyroidism affects 1 in 6 people.

Other types of thyroid disease also influence weight gain. Pseudohypoparathyroidism, also called Martin-Albright Syndrome, is a genetic disorder that is caused by a lack of response to parathyroid hormone. It's a rare cause of pediatric obesity. People with pseudohypoparathyroidism may also have abnormally round faces, thick short bodies, unusually short fourth fingers, and mental retardation. Symptoms include headaches, weakness, and fatigue, lack of energy, blurred vision, and hypersensitivity to light.

Parathyroid hormone helps regulate calcium and phosphate levels in the blood. In pseudohypoparathyroidism, the hormone is adequately synthesized, but the kidneys are resistant to it.

Treatment for pseudohypoparathyroidism consists of taking calcium and vitamin D supplements. If you think you or your child may have this condition, it's important to see a physician.

POLYCYSTIC OVARY SYNDROME (PCOS)

THE MISUNDERSTOOD DISEASE

An estimated 5% to 8% of women of childbearing age have PCOS. It is a poorly understood complex disorder, which can cause a wide range of potentially serious symptoms, including obesity and infertility. Women with PCOS also have an increased risk of heart disease and diabetes.

PCOS often affects multiple endocrine glands, including the thyroid, pancreas, and adrenals. In many patients, androgen excess results in oily skin, acne, and facial hair.

Women with PCOS often become insulin resistant. Insulin, produced by the pancreas, helps cells utilize glucose for energy.

In insulin resistance, the body's muscle, fat and liver cells can't use insulin properly and excess

Women with PCOS also have an increased risk of heart disease and diabetes.

sugars build up in the bloodstream. If untreated, women with PCOS have a 10% to 20% increased risk of developing type 2 diabetes by the time they reach middle age.

PCOS can lead to serious health problems such as heart disease, endometrial cancer, pregnancy complications, and hypertensive disorders. A study conducted in Sweden found that women with PCOS are seven times more likely to suffer heart attacks in their 40s or 50s as compared to women the same age without PCOS.

One of the most frustrating symptoms of PCOS is weight gain. Women with PCOS are more apt to gain weight and have more trouble losing weight than the average woman, and nearly half of PCOS patients are overweight.

Fat distribution in women with PCOS tends to occur around the abdomen, resulting in an "apple figure"—the most dangerous type of fat. It can lead to the development of high cholesterol, heart disease and hypertension.

Weight gain is often associated with a worsening of PCOS symptoms such as hirsutism, irregular menstrual periods, and infertility. Yet weight loss of just 5% of body weight can improve these symptoms.

Metformin (Glucophage), a diabetes medication, may facilitate weight loss, along with diet and exercise. Some studies have found that metformin can help regulate insulin levels and triglycerides, alleviate acne, and reduce facial hair.

To help regulate hormones, some women with PCOS may be placed on birth control pills. Because responses to the birth control pill can be highly individual, only some women respond well to this medication.

A recent study by researchers at Pennsylvania State University published in *Fertility and Sterility* tied high protein, low-carb diets to weight loss as well as improved menstrual regularity, lipid profiles, and insulin resistance in obese women with PCOS. Low carb diets, modified-carb diets, and

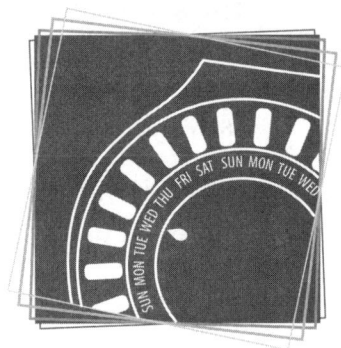

insulin-regulating diets may be helpful for weight loss in PCOS. The reason? These diets reduce sugar consumption, which slows down unhealthy fat storage.

Physical activity is just as important as dietary improvements—for control of insulin resistance as well as weight loss. Any increase in activity can help the body utilize more insulin. Most physicians recommend at least 30 minutes of exercise three times a week. Daily exercise is important if weight loss is a goal.

FAT & CUSHING'S SYNDROME

Cushing's disease, also called hypercortisolism, is a rare endocrine disorder that occurs when the adrenal glands produce too much cortisol, a stress hormone. Cushing's syndrome can also be caused by some drugs like corticosteroids, used to treat inflammatory diseases such as lupus and rheumatoid arthritis. A tumor of the pituitary gland, adrenal adenomas, or certain types of malignancies in other parts of the body can also cause the production of too much cortisol.

Excess cortisol causes fat accumulation in the face, abdomen, and upper back, often producing a round "moon face" and "buffalo hump," while the arms and legs usually remain slender. Other symptoms include muscle wasting and weakness, thin skin, poor wound healing, easy bruising, purple "stretch marks" on the abdomen, menstrual irregularities, high blood pressure, and hair loss.

Although it may not be possible to prevent weight gain in Cushing's Syndrome, diet modification can help minimize the extra pounds, and a low-sodium diet may be helpful in preventing excess fluid retention.

It is possible to cure or treat Cushing's syndrome. If the illness is caused by a pituitary tumor, surgery or radiotherapy may be curative.

DISABILITIES & WEIGHT GAIN: WHAT'S THE CONNECTION?

Obesity and disabilities are often linked. In a study published in the January/February 2004 issue of *Health Affairs*, researchers reported that the number of people with disabilities between age 30 and 49 rose more than 50% from 1984 to 2000. According to the researchers, the leading causes of disability are musculoskeletal problems, such as chronic back pain. People with disabilities are more likely to suffer from fatigue, pain and movement disorders that make it difficult to exercise, and easier to gain weight.

MULTIPLE SCLEROSIS (MS)

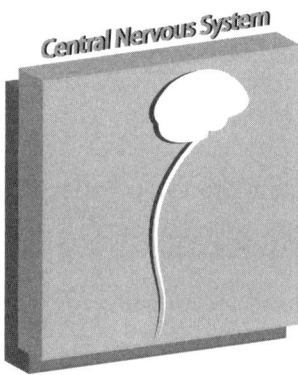
Central Nervous System

MS is a chronic demyelinating disease of the central nervous system. Mobility and physical activity are often severely restricted by the disease, and the result can sometimes be weight gain. Carrying around extra pounds can also *increase* fatigue and put a strain on respiratory and circulatory systems, making it more difficult to exercise and maintain a healthy weight. Certain kinds of fatigue (neuromuscular, depression-related, and MS lassitude) are common among MS patients.

Exercise can alleviate feelings of fatigue and depression, and help maintain bowel and bladder function, as well as a healthy weight. Inactivity can lead to an increased risk of coronary heart disease, muscle weakness, bone loss and respiratory problems. Research shows that MS patients who exercise regularly have better cardiovascular fitness, improved strength, better bladder and bowel function, less fatigue and depression, and an increased interest in social activities.

The Multiple Sclerosis Society recommends an exercise program that is tailored to the patient's capabilities. Lifting weights helps develop strength and maintain good bone mineral density. Gentle activities such as yoga and stretching can help improve flexibility. Patients with MS should avoid exercising during the hottest part of the day and drink plenty of water to avoid overheating.

FIBROMYALGIA SYNDROME (FMS)

FMS is a common disorder characterized by pain throughout the body, fatigue, difficulty sleeping, and increased pain sensitivity to pressure. Seven to ten million Americans suffer from FMS. It affects many more women than men, and most problems begin when patients are in their 40s and 50s.

A study published in the *Scandinavian Journal of Rheumatology* was the first to suggest the link

Seven to ten million Americans suffer from FMS.

between FMS and obesity. Researchers evaluated 211 women with FMS and divided them into groups based on their BMI. FMS symptoms were rated over a month's time. The researchers found that a majority of FMS patients are overweight due in part to physical inactivity. Women with higher BMIs also had more severe FMS symptoms, especially fatigue and tender points. The authors propose that weight loss by FMS patients may improve function and possibly fatigue.

There is evidence that regular exercise is beneficial for FMS patients. However, exercise is not an easy chore for FMS patients, because of the muscle pain and post-exertional fatigue they experience. The most popular and easiest types of exercise for FMS patients are walking, riding a stationary bike, or aquatic therapy. High impact exercises such as jogging, basketball, and aerobics should be avoided.

There is currently no cure for FMS. Drugs such as aspirin, non-steroidal anti-inflammatories

(NSAIDs), such as ibuprofen, and cortisone are not particularly helpful for reducing the musculoskeletal pain. Opioids, such as codeine, hydrocodone, and oxycodone, may provide some pain relief, but FMS patients appear to be very sensitive to the side effects of these medications, and addiction can be problematic. Normalizing sleep architecture with low doses of non-benzodiazepine hypnotics such as *zolpidem* (Ambien) or *zaleplon* (Sonata) often affords significant relief. Another useful adjunct is tender point injection. *Pregabalin* (Lyrica), *milnacipran* (Savella), and *duloxetine* (Cymbalta) are sometimes useful in these patients.

There is currently no cure for FMS.

CHRONIC FATIGUE SYNDROME (CFS)

CFS is an illness characterized by prolonged debilitating fatigue and multiple symptoms such as headache, recurrent sore throat, muscle and joint pain, and difficulty with memory and concentration. The condition is also called myalgic encephalomyelitis, post viral fatigue syndrome, and chronic fatigue and immune dysfunction syndrome. Profound fatigue, the primary symptom of this disorder, can come on suddenly or gradually. CFS symptoms linger for at least six months and often for years.

Gentle, regular exercise can lessen body aches and joint and muscle pain, increase energy, and control weight gain. When exercising, proceeding with caution is key, however. Although physical activity and exercise can help with symptom relief, in some cases it can actually exacerbate symptoms. Restoring normal sleep architecture is essential in relieving symptoms. A careful medical evaluation to rule out other illnesses is essential as well.

STROKE

Stroke is the leading cause of disability in older Americans. Symptoms of stroke include behavior changes, memory loss, confusion, depression, paralysis, sudden laughing or crying, communication problems, and difficulty performing daily tasks, such as dressing and grooming.

A person may become inactive due to a stroke, and as a result may gain weight. Patients may then find it even more difficult to exercise. This inactivity is cause for concern, because there is mounting evidence that exercise is very beneficial for stroke patients. According to a small study published in *Stroke*, stroke survivors who completed an in-hospital rehabilitation program followed by therapist-supervised physical therapy significantly improved their endurance, balance, and walking ability.

An aggressive home-based exercise program can improve physical outcomes for stroke patients. The program should incorporate strength, balance, endurance, and upper extremity exercises into a comprehensive stroke recovery protocol.

CONGESTIVE HEART FAILURE & ASTHMA

An estimated five million Americans have congestive heart failure, and it is one of the leading causes of hospital admissions. Congestive heart failure occurs when the heart cannot pump enough blood to meet the requirements of the body. As the heart deteriorates, excess fluid begins to accumulate in different parts of the body, causing edema and weight gain. Other symptoms include shortness of breath, tiredness, weakness, loss of appetite, and cough. Heart failure is debilitating and can cause people to give up many of the activities they enjoy. Recent research demonstrates that obesity elevates the risk for diastolic dysfunction that often leads to heart failure.

Treatment of congestive heart failure includes medication and lifestyle changes such as avoiding salt, alcohol, and tobacco and excess fluid intake, losing weight, and exercising regularly. Recent studies suggest that exercise can help weight loss efforts in congestive heart failure patients.

As a general rule, the American Heart Association recommends that people with heart failure stay active. Exercise can improve symptoms, reduce stress, and increase energy levels. Regular exercises such as walking or biking will help increase muscle tone and strength, taking some of the workload off the heart and reducing symptoms as a result. However, it is important

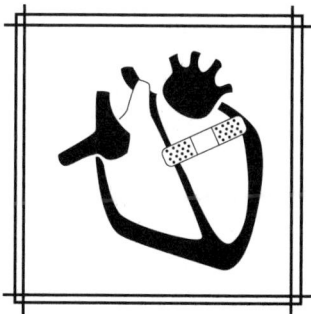

to note that exercise must be balanced with rest and relaxation to accommodate symptoms of fatigue.

In addition to exercise, physicians recommend a low-salt diet (2.4 grams per day) to help limit fluid retention. Certain medications such as beta-blockers, diuretics, ACE inhibitors, and ARBs (angiotensin II receptor blockers) can reduce symptoms and slow the progression of the disease.

A thorough medical examination is the first step before beginning any kind of exercise program. A period of low-level aerobic activity will prepare the body for higher-intensity activities.

Patients with asthma should take extra time to warm up before exercising. Exercise should be done toward the lower end of the target heart rate. Walking and swimming are good options because they are low-intensity in nature, and can be done for longer periods of time. Asthmatics should avoid exercising in polluted environments or in cold or dry air, and a long cool-down period following exercise will help prevent an asthma attack immediately after a workout.

MEDICATIONS: WHICH CAUSE WEIGHT GAIN?

Weight gain is a common side effect of many prescribed drugs. These include drugs taken for diabetes, hypertension, gastric reflux and heartburn, and depression and other psychiatric disorders. However, even those medications that list weight gain as a side effect may not necessarily cause a *large* weight gain. And in some cases it may be years before the weight gain emerges.

Antidepressants are among the medications that cause persistent and problematic weight gain—particularly tricyclic antidepressants. Often the excessive weight gain produced by tricyclic antidepressants results in medication noncompliance.

A review study published in the *Primary Care Companion to the Journal of Clinical Psychiatry,* found that weight gain may be common even among patients on long-term therapy with other types of antidepressants—the SSRIs, such as *fluoxetine* (Prozac) and *sertraline* (Zoloft). Though patients tend to lose weight in the first six months of taking SSRIs, additional weight gain has been reported with long-term use.

CHAPTER 3

Uncontrolled studies have shown mean weight gain of patients on SSRIs ranging from 15 to 24 pounds after 6 to 12 months of therapy.

Though patients tend to lose weight in the first six months of taking SSRIs, additional weight gain has been reported with long-term use.

Some of the top-selling medications that cause weight gain include heartburn drugs such as *esomeprazole magnesium* (Nexium) and *lansoprazole* (Prevacid), and multiple diabetes drugs. Antihistamines such as *loratadine* (Claritin, Claritin RediTabs, Alavert) and high blood pressure medications can all cause weight gain.

Weight gain is also a well-known side effect of steroids like prednisone. Weight gain may be caused by a class of drugs called second generation antipsychotics (SGAs), such as *olanzapine* (Zyprexa), a drug commonly used for bipolar disorder.

These drugs work by altering levels of hormones and neuropeptides, and even a slight change in the levels have an effect on appetite and satiety. Some

SGAs can cause rapid weight gain and predispose patients to pre-diabetes.

Other medications that sometimes affect weight are hormone replacement therapy and oral contraceptives, which can cause fluid retention and increased appetite.

One of the major adverse effects of *valproate*, a drug widely used for treating epilepsy and bipolar disorder, is weight gain. A study published in *Epilepsy Research*, compared the effects of *valproate* and *lamotrigine*, another anti-seizure drug, on hormone and fat levels, prevalence of menstrual disorders, and body weight. Researchers found that compared with those taking *lamotrigine*, women on *valproate* gained more weight and had higher androgen levels, as well as more problems with their menstrual cycles. According to the study, *valproate*-induced weight gain may play a pivotal role in causing hormone and lipid abnormalities in women with epilepsy. Thus *lamotrigine* may be a better choice for some women with epilepsy, especially those with reproductive problems or lipid abnormalities.

It is important to keep in mind that while these drugs may cause an increase in weight, they have helped millions of people manage their symptoms. Other therapeutic options may exist, however. If there are no good alternatives, talk with your doctor about ways to limit weight gain while you're taking the medication.

...while these drugs may cause an increase in weight, they have helped millions of people manage their symptoms.

Drugs that may cause weight gain include:

ANTIDEPRESSANTS

Amitriptyline (Elavil, Endep)
Desipramine (Norpramin, Pertofrane)
Mirtazapine (Remeron)
Nortriptyline (Aventyl, Pamelor)
Paroxetine (Paxil)
Sertraline (Zoloft)
Trazodone (Desyrel)

ANTI-ESTROGENS

Danazol (Danocrine)
Leuprolide acetate (Lupron)

ANTIHISTAMINES

Chlorpheniramine (Alermine, Chlor-Trimeton)
Diphenhydramine (Benadryl, Sominex Formula)
Loratadine (Claritin tablets, syrup)

BLOOD PRESSURE MEDICATIONS

Beta-blockers: *acebutolol* (Sectral), *atenolol* (Tenormin), *propranolol* (Inderal)
Prazosin (Minipress)
Terazosin (Hytrin)

CORTICOSTEROIDS

Betamethasone (Diprolene, Diprosine, Valisone, Selstoject)
Dexamethasone (Decadron, Hexadrol, TobraDex, etc.)
Methylprednisolone (Depopred, Medrol)
Prednisone (Deltasone, Meticorten, Prednicen-M)

DIABETES MEDICATIONS

Insulin
Glipizide (Glucotrol)
Glyburide (Diabeta)
Nateglinide (Starlix)
Pioglitazone (Actos)
Repaglinide (Prandin)

HORMONE REPLACEMENT THERAPY

Estrogen medications such as Premarin; progestins

NONSTEROIDAL ANTI-INFLAMMATORY DRUGS (NSAIDs)

These drugs may cause weight gain due to sodium retention.

Ibuprofen (Advil, Motrin, etc)

Naproxen (Naprosyn, Anaprox)

OTHER PSYCHIATRIC MEDICATIONS

Clorpromazine (Thorazine)

Lithium (Eskalith, Lithobid, Lithonate)

Olanzapine (Zyprexa)

Perphenazine (Etrafon, Triavil, Trilafon, and others that combine *perphenazine* and *amitriptyline*)

Quetiapine (Seroquel)

Valproate (Depakene, Depakote, Depacon)

SLEEP AIDS

Chlordiazepoxide (Librium)

Diazepam (Valium)

Flurazepam (Dalmane)

Temazepam (Restoril)

Zolpidem (Ambien)

MOST ANTICONVULSANTS

Obesity in children is now an epidemic in the United States. Children whose parents are overweight may be genetically predisposed to weight problems, but genetics isn't the only reason; there's another culprit—inactivity. About half of children and adolescents aged 8 to 16 watch three to five hours of TV every day. Those children who watch the most TV have the highest incidence of obesity. Today, even more time is spent in front of computers and smartphones.

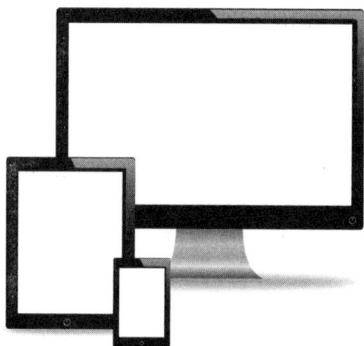

Emerging evidence shows that obese children and adolescents have increased risk of high cholesterol and blood pressure, sleep apnea, orthopedic problems, liver disease, asthma, and type 2 diabetes. According to researchers at the State University of New York at Buffalo, a healthier family lifestyle can improve a child's BMI.

The researchers evaluated 42 children aged 8 to 12 years who attended a pediatric obesity clinic with their parents. They participated in a

Quick Tips

Weight Loss in Children: Advice for Parents

- Avoid pre-prepared and sugared foods when possible.
- Limit the amount of high-calorie foods kept in the home.
- Provide a healthy diet, with 30% or fewer calories derived from fat.
- Provide ample fiber in the child's diet.
- Skim milk may safely replace whole milk at two years of age.
- Do not provide food for comfort or as a reward.
- Do not offer sweets in exchange for a finished meal.
- Limit amount of television viewing and computer time.
- Encourage active play.
- Establish regular family activities such as walks, ball games, and other outdoor activities.

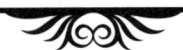

two-year family-based weight control program, which included only families with parents with high BMIs. The researchers found that weight loss in parents was associated with weight loss in children; children of parents who lost the most weight were more likely to lose weight too.

So parents should make physical fitness and healthy eating a family priority.

GETTING RID OF PREGNANCY POUNDS

After giving birth most women want to return to their pre-pregnancy weight as soon as possible. For some women this weight loss may take up to a year. Others will never regain their shape, however, and some women will even gain weight. Many women find it difficult to lose their pregnancy weight for a wide range of reasons, from genetics to time restraints.

Although there are few studies on weight reduction programs for postpartum weight loss, calorie restriction, exercise, or both have been shown to be effective. Restricting the diet to 1,800 kcal per day for breast-feeding women has been shown to be safe while still achieving weight loss.

Trying to lose weight while breastfeeding is still a controversial subject, however. Some research indicates that exercising while breastfeeding may impair the quantity and quality of milk. Another issue is the level of intensity at which a lactating woman exercises. Infants are less accepting of breast milk 30 minutes after high-intensity exercise. Studies published in the *Annals of Behavioral Medicine and Pediatrics* in 2002 and 2003, however, show that aerobic exercise without dieting doesn't affect breast-milk volume or concentration.

Research and clinical experience demonstrate that if new mothers don't lose the pregnancy weight within six months of giving birth, they may never lose it.

A review study published in the *Annals of Behavioral Medicine* in 2003 evaluated postpartum weight retention in women. The study turned up several interesting findings. Weight gain after giving birth is highly individual, and women who had higher weights before getting pregnant were at high risk for retaining their weight gain postpartum. Retaining weight gain also seems particularly prevalent among minority women. The study found that African American women retained twice as much weight after

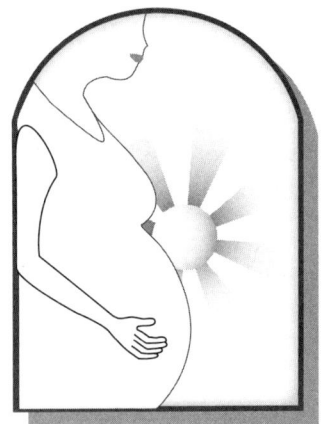

...women who had higher weights before getting pregnant were at high risk for retaining their weight gain postpartum.

pregnancy as white women did.

Weight loss programs that integrate increased physical activity with dietary changes such as calorie restriction and eating low-fat foods are effective in producing weight loss in women after pregnancy. Behavioral weight loss techniques such as self-monitoring (for instance, keeping track of the foods you eat) are also helpful.

MENOPAUSE: AVOIDING THOSE EXTRA POUNDS

It's still open to debate what role, if any, menopause plays in midlife weight gain. Hormonal changes that occur during menopause may contribute to weight gain. Yet some experts feel it's not menopause, but the lifestyle changes women go through as they age that cause weight gain. Our metabolic rate declines about 5% per decade beginning in our 20s.

Quick Tips
Staying Healthy during Menopause

- Avoid foods that increase the likelihood of hot flashes such as alcohol, caffeine, and spicy foods.

- Bone up on calcium. It is especially important to have adequate levels of calcium in your diet. After age 50, women require 1,200 mg of calcium and 800 IU of vitamin D_3 per day to prevent bone loss and possibly reduce the risk of fractures. Excessive consumption of calcium supplements may lead to calcium deposition in arteries.

- Stay active. During menopause, the body's metabolism slows down, making it harder to keep weight off. In addition to increasing your activity level to burn more calories, exercise protects the muscle mass you already have and helps the body to burn more calories. Experts recommend 30 to 60 minutes of aerobic exercise most days of the week. Strength training can help build muscle and burn calories more efficiently.

- Eat lots of fruit and vegetables. They contain heart-healthy antioxidants, are low in calories, and contribute fiber.

- Be more conscious of portion sizes, and reduce your intake of saturated fats.

- Cut out sodas and sugar-laden beverages.

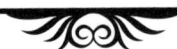

Many women gain an average of 10 pounds during menopause, but this amount of weight gain is not inevitable. A healthy lifestyle can compensate for weight challenges brought about by menopause. Good nutrition can help reduce hot flashes, keep bones strong, keep the heart healthy and help manage weight and energy levels.

Menopausal women may be more susceptible to weight gain because symptoms such as joint aches and pains (commonly associated with menopause) may temporarily make exercise uncomfortable. Overweight postmenopausal women are at increased risk for hypertension, diabetes, and coronary artery disease, but weight loss can significantly decrease many of these risk factors, as well as helping to alleviate the symptoms of menopause.

WEIGHT LOSS IN SENIORS

Even in the elderly, exercise keeps people limber, reduces muscle atrophy, keeps lungs in better condition and boosts energy. People approaching their golden years should choose a sensible diet that's high in nutrition. Protein is especially important because as the body ages, it loses lean muscle mass.

As well as weight gain, disease-related weight loss can be a problem in the elderly. Many elderly patients experience a physiologic weight loss of 1–2 pounds per year beginning around age 74.

A study conducted at the Yale University School of Medicine analyzed the relationship between physical activity and weight change in the elderly. The researchers found that among frail people older than 65 years, even modest levels of physical activity can ease the rate of aging and disease-related weight loss.

THE BOTTOM LINE

Many of us are concerned about our weight, and it's often a frustrating task to achieve the weight loss we want.

Yet in some cases, our inability to lose the weight may be aggravated by illness or life changes that are beyond our control—or medications we may need for our health. So before you blame yourself for your lack of willpower, check with your doctor, and explain your concerns. Proper diagnosis and treatment of underlying medical conditions, appropriate medication changes, and guidance with lifestyle may improve weight loss efforts.

Chapter 4

fad diets & popular weight loss plans: which ones work?

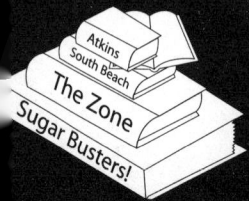

"Going on a diet inherently implies that, at some point, you're going to go off the diet."

~ Wise Old Geriatrician

Fad diets have always appealed to people as an easy way to lose weight. Today's fad diets range from the cabbage soup and South Beach diet to low fat veggie weight loss plans. Why are fad diets popular? They generally promise, and in many cases result in, rapid weight loss. Yet they provide a temporary solution to being overweight, rather than promoting permanent changes in nutrition and lifestyle—healthy habits that can be maintained for a lifetime. After all, how long can you stand to eat cabbage soup to keep the pounds off?

It may be easier, at first, to lose weight on a fad diet. Yet in the long run you're better off with a realistic healthy eating plan that provides you with a full range of nutrients and increased energy, as well as a smaller waistline.

Every day, we're bombarded with ads for the newest weight loss products, all promising trim bodies and a quick fix for the overweight and obese. An increasing number of diet gurus are promoting their diet plans and supplements as the best way to drop pounds and maintain weight loss.

Some of these diets seem far-fetched—at least on the surface. One popular best-selling book, for instance, discourages eating turkey sandwiches, because they put a strain on your digestive system. Another advises arranging the food on your plate by volume so that you eat equal amounts of sloppy Joe meat, asparagus with hollandaise sauce, and hot cherry cobbler a la mode.

Another craze in weight loss is the low-carb diet. These weight loss plans range from the steak and cheesecake Atkins diet to the more healthy South Beach and Zone diets. Proponents say they work effectively to reduce weight as well as risk of cardiovascular disease.

Low-carbohydrate foods such as those prescribed in the Atkins and South Beach diets were popular several years ago. A wave of low-carb products hit the marketplace, including low-carb bread, energy bars, cookies, and even low-carb beer. Subway announced the addition of two low-carb sandwiches to their offerings. The Coca-Cola Company added a low-carb version of Coke to their product line.

Some of today's low-carb diets have gained a smattering of scientific support as effective ways to lose weight, and can decrease some risk factors for chronic illnesses such as heart disease and diabetes. Proponents claim these diets are easier to stick to than low-fat diets, and result in quick weight loss without hunger pangs.

According to low-carb proponents, carbohydrates are unhealthy because they provide a quick, unsustained, energy boost. Carbohydrates raise insulin levels, resulting in low blood sugar levels and increased food cravings. The result is weight gain and obesity.

Yet low-carb diets have not been proven in large studies for either effective *long-term* weight loss or reduction of chronic disease risk. There is also evidence to suggest that these diets may

CHAPTER 4

Quick Tips

Easy Ways to Cook Healthy

- Bake, broil, roast, steam or microwave food instead of frying it.

- If food must be fried, use a small amount of canola or olive oil or a nonstick cooking spray; limit butter or margarine.

- Choose lean cuts of red meat and remove all visible fat before cooking.

- Removing the skin from poultry before cooking reduces fat by 25%.

- Season food with herbs, spices, and lemon juice rather than butter and salt.

- Substitute real fruit juices for sugar in recipes

- Substitute applesauce for butter, margarine, or shortening in recipes.

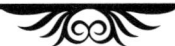

be unhealthy in the long run since they deprive the body of many of the nutrients found in carbohydrates. They also eliminate or limit many unquestionably healthy foods, such as fruits and starchy vegetables.

Eating fewer than 20 grams of carbohydrates a day can lead to the buildup of ketones (partially broken-down fats) in the blood. A buildup of ketones (called ketosis) can cause high levels of uric acid, which is a risk factor for gout and kidney stones.

According to the American Heart Association, "Diets low in carbohydrates are likely to lack sufficient amounts of essential nutrients found in plant foods that promote good health. People following these diets may not get enough vitamins, minerals, and fiber to avoid blood chemistry imbalances, constipation, and other health problems."

THE SCOOP ON LOW-CARB DIETS

The popularity of low-carbohydrate diets increased following the publication of *Dr. Atkins' New Diet Revolution*, which was on the New York Times bestseller list for five years.

The idea of a low-carb diet is not new. A diet similar to the Atkins diet was first proposed by William Banting, an undertaker, in 1863, based on his discussions with a surgeon friend. His basic idea was that diets high in protein and low in carbohydrates promote the metabolism of fat

CHAPTER 4

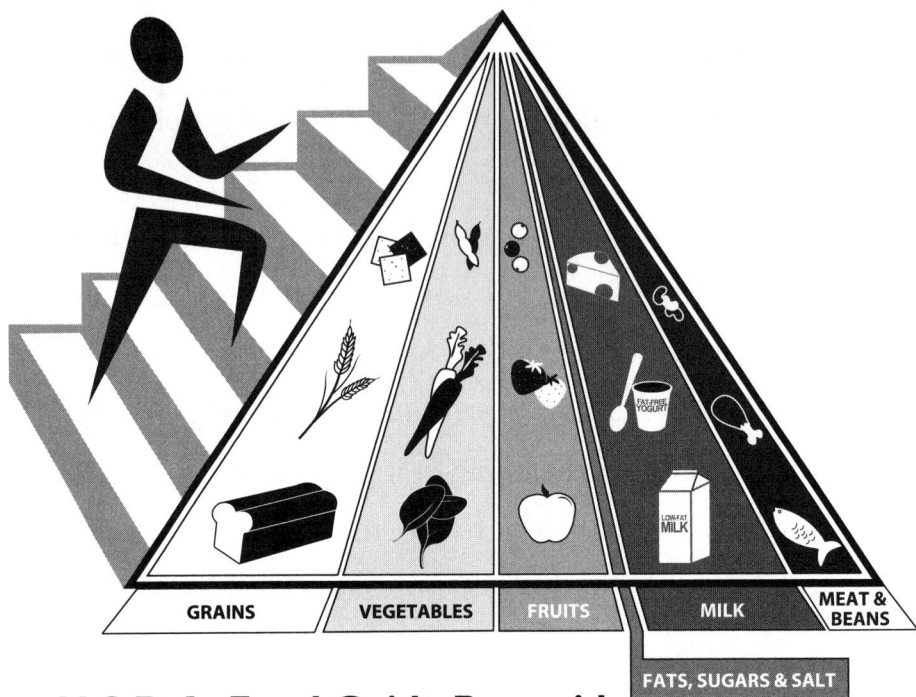

U.S.D.A. Food Guide Pyramid

U.S. Department of Agriculture and the U.S. Department of Health and Human Services

GRAINS – Eat 6 oz. every day, including 3 oz. from whole-grain foods.

VEGETABLES – Eat 2½ cups every day. Vary your veggies. Eat more dark green and orange veggies, and more dry beans and peas.

FRUITS – Eat 2 cups every day. Choose fresh, frozen, canned or dried fruit. Go easy on fruit juices.

MILK – Get enough calcium-rich foods. Go low-fat or fat-free when you choose milk or yogurt products.

MEAT & BEANS – Choose low-fat or lean meats and poultry. Bake, broil or grill meats, poultry and fish. Vary your protein—try more fish, beans, peas, nuts, and seeds.

Know the limits on **FATS, SUGARS,** and **SALT** (sodium)
- Make most of your fat sources from fish, nuts, and vegetable oils.
- Limit solid fats like butter, stick margarine, shortening, and lard, as well as foods that contain these.
- Check the Nutrition Facts label to keep saturated fats, trans fats, and sodium low.
- Choose food and beverages low in added sugars. Added sugars contribute calories with few, if any, nutrients.

WEIGHT PERFECT

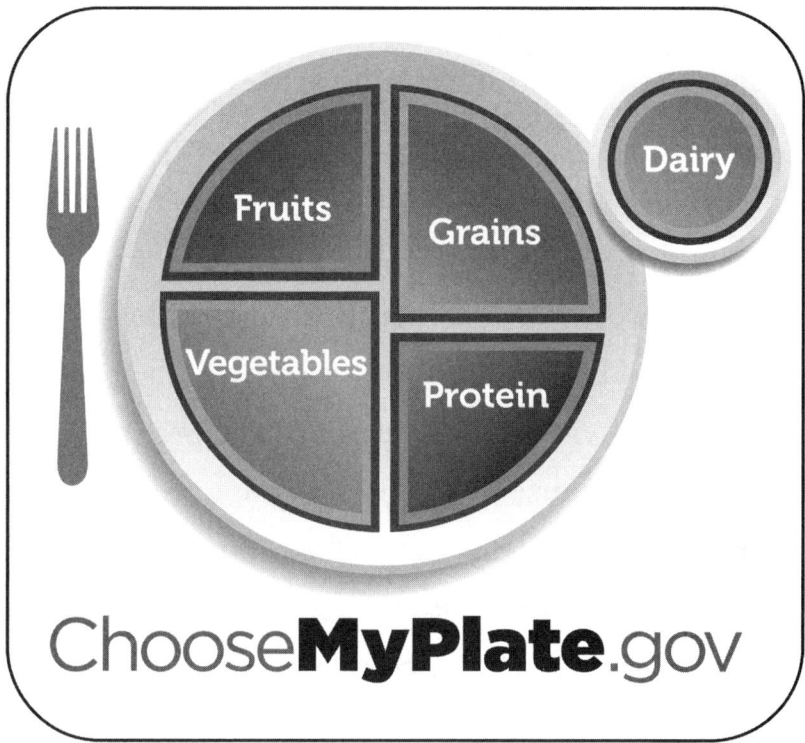

ChooseMyPlate.gov

U.S.D.A. MyPlate

MyPlate is the U.S. Department of Agriculture's food guidance icon. It is a visual cue that identifies the five (5) basic food groups from which consumers can choose to build a healthy plate at mealtimes. It encourages healthy food choices and healthy eating habits, consistent with the *2010 Dietary Guidelines for Americans*.

For more information, go to *http://www.choosemyplate.gov*.

tissue when carbohydrates are not available as an energy source, resulting in rapid weight loss with no adverse effects.

Consumption of too many refined carbs can make it more difficult to control weight because these carbs are very rapidly absorbed, leading to high blood sugar levels followed by high surges of insulin. After two or three hours, the large amounts of insulin cause the blood sugar levels to drop abruptly, sometimes even below normal levels. When this happens, hunger strikes—often leading to snacking and increased calorie intake.

High amounts of carbs also reduce the levels of HDL cholesterol in the blood (the good cholesterol). Low HDL is one risk factor for heart disease.

In one study on low-carb diets, published in the *Annals of Internal Medicine* in 2004, researchers evaluated the health effects of a low-carb diet versus one in which subjects reduced their calorie intake by 500 calories per day. Those on the low carb diet lost the same amount of weight as those on the low calorie diet after one year. However, people on the low-carb diet showed bigger drops in triglyceride levels and had higher HDL levels.

Carbohydrates & the Glycemic Index

High-glycemic		Low-glycemic	
• Potatoes	• Bananas	• Most legumes	• Whole fruits
• White bread	• White rice	• Whole wheat	• Oats
• French fries	• White spaghetti	• Bran	• Brown rice
• Soft drinks	• Sugar	• Bulgur	• Barley
• Refined breakfast cereals		• Whole-grain breakfast cereals	• Couscous

Source: Nutrition Source, Harvard School of Public Health.

The researchers acknowledged, however, that their conclusions were limited by a high dropout rate (34%) for both diets.

Many researchers agree that the type of carbs consumed is quite important. Thus it's helpful to replace highly refined starches, such as white bread and white rice, with the whole grain versions of these foods.

CHAPTER 4

LOW-CARB DIETS: HOW THEY WORK

What's involved in following a low-carb diet?

Here's a look at the pros and cons of some of the more popular low-carb eating plans.

The Atkins program is a high-protein diet that allows 20 grams of carbohydrates at the start. The diet works by inducing a state of ketosis. In ketosis, the body is forced to burn fat when carbohydrates are limited.

Carbohydrates are severely restricted during the first two weeks in the Atkins diet, and a large initial weight loss occurs. However, this rapid decrease in weight occurs primarily because of fluid loss. Then a limited amount of carbohydrates are slowly reintroduced into the diet.

Pros:

∾ Does result in rapid weight loss

∾ Provides a feeling of satiety

∾ Allows abundant consumption of protein and fats

Cons:

∾ There is debate about whether high consumption of animal protein leads to increased cholesterol levels and heart disease.

∾ There is some dispute about whether or not ketosis is damaging to the body (especially the liver) long-term.

Quick Tip

Beware of these "Low-Carb" Foods

Some of the health food products in the grocery aisles—touted as "low-carb"—are actually loaded with carbs. Energy bars and low-carb cookies are labeled as "sugar free" when they actually contain as much as 25 grams of sugar alcohols. Though this claim isn't exactly false, it is misleading.

Sugar alcohols are sugar substitutes that contain carbs. They can also cause a significant rise in blood sugar levels—though a much slower and smaller rise than regular refined sugar. These products also have a laxative effect, resulting in diarrhea, gas and bloating. So, when shopping for low-carb products, read labels: Choose foods that contain low amounts of sugar as well as sugar alcohols.

- There is also debate as to whether the body burns lean muscle mass for fuel, and not just fat, on a low-carb diet.
- Many of the high-protein foods included in the program are high in saturated fat and low in vitamins and minerals.
- There is a lack of fiber in the diet.
- The first phase has a high drop-out rate, as some people find it difficult to entirely give up carbohydrates.
- The program does not promote balanced eating.

The South Beach Diet was developed in 1999 by Dr. Arthur Agatston, a Florida-based cardiologist, in an effort to help his patients lose weight. It is similar to the Atkins diet, but it differentiates between "good" (complex) and "bad" (simple) carbs and "good" (monounsaturated) and "bad" (saturated) fats. It provides daily guidance for balanced meals and snacks. Like the Atkins plan, it severely restricts carbohydrates in the beginning weeks of the diet, but complex carbohydrates are then slowly reintroduced.

Pros:

∾ It is considered scientifically sound and is recommended by Lawrence Cheskin, M.D., director of the Weight Management Center at Johns Hopkins Hospital.

∾ It differentiates between "good" and "bad" carbs and fats.

∾ It improves cholesterol and insulin levels.

∾ It promotes a balance between major food groups, rather than eliminating some of them, and provides practical eating patterns.

∾ It has a low drop-out rate.

Quick Tips

Healthful Grocery Shopping

- Shop the outside aisles, which contain healthy foods like fruit, vegetables, chicken, and fish.

- Read food labels and be aware of high fat and sugar content.

- Never shop for food when you are hungry.

- Make a grocery list and stick to it. Do not buy on impulse.

- Avoid processed meats like bacon, sausage, and packaged cold cuts, as they are high in fat and salt.

- Do not buy unhealthy or fattening foods—if they are not in your house, you will be less tempted to eat them.

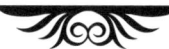

Cons:

ᴄᴠ Much of the initial weight loss may just be water loss caused by cutting out carbs.

ᴄᴠ It is not recommended for people with kidney problems.

ᴄᴠ Vegetarians would find it difficult to follow the menus as the regimen is meat oriented.

THE ZONE

The Zone diet is a low-carbohydrate diet made up of 40% protein, 30% carbohydrates, and

Quick Tips

Some tips for eating at fast food restaurants:

- Choose chicken that's grilled, not fried.

- Hold the mayo, or ask for a low-fat or non-fat version. Mustard can also be a good choice for a sandwich spread.

- Ask for light or fat-free salad dressings. Or use the regular sparingly.

- Skip the fries.

- Order veggie pizza—it almost always has less total fat than any other kind.

Source: Environmental Nutrition newsletter

30% fats created by Barry Sears, Ph.D. It claims to regulate the body's blood sugar levels and insulin production, thus maximizing fat loss. It allows proteins and some fats. Carbohydrates in the form of vegetables and fruits, rich in fiber, can also be included in meals. Protein is eaten at every meal and snack, and the amount of carbohydrates consumed should be twice the amount of protein. Complex carbohydrates are favored, and simple carbs should only be eaten in small quantities.

Pros:

∾ The diet includes abundant amounts of fruits and low-starch vegetables.

∾ It is low in saturated fats.

∾ Simple carbohydrates are restricted.

∾ Adherents experience a steady weight loss if it is followed exactly.

Cons:

∾ Achieving the exact 40-30-30 ratio required can be quite complicated.

∾ Restricted calorie intake (800 to 1,200 calories) can make following the diet difficult.

∾ The diet is low in whole grains.

∾ The prepackaged Zone products are expensive.

∾ It provides only a short-term solution to weight loss, because the diet is based on a very low caloric intake that is difficult to sustain.

Dr. Phil's Ultimate Weight Solution

Phil McGraw, Ph.D., is a psychologist who rose to fame as a motivational guru on Oprah, and now has his own spin-off show. His book, *The Ultimate Weight Solution: The 7 Keys to Weight Loss Freedom,* is primarily a self-help book that recommends behavioral changes such as portion control, choosing healthy foods, and sitting down to meals. The personalized meals include complex carbohydrates, fruits and vegetables, and lean protein and healthy fats. There is also a section concerning supplements that aid weight loss according to body type, but there is no scientific evidence supporting their efficacy.

Pros:

∾ Promotes healthy eating

∾ Encourages behavior modification with regard to eating

Cons:

∾ Approach to lifestyle changes is somewhat oversimplified

∾ The supplements discussed have no particular bearing on weight loss or control.

SUGAR BUSTERS!

The Sugar Busters Diet first appeared in the 1995 book, *Sugar Busters!*, which was written by three physicians and the CEO of a Fortune 500 company. It is based on the theory that sugar is toxic and when consumed causes an increase in insulin, which in turn encourages weight gain. All refined

Good Weight Loss Foods

Some types of foods actually help you lose those unwanted pounds.

Calcium: Studies show that people who take in the most calcium (from food sources, rather than supplements) are more likely to be successful at weight loss, and less likely to gain weight over the long-term.

Fiber: Fruits, vegetables and whole grains fill you up because of the large amounts of fiber they contain. Thus, you're less likely to overindulge in junk foods with lots of fat and sugar.

A study published in the *American Journal of Clinical Nutrition* in 2004 showed that people who increased their intake of whole fruits and low-fat milk over six years had a significantly reduced risk of gaining weight.

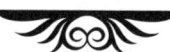

sugar is eliminated, and foods with a high glycemic index (a measure of food's effect on raising blood sugar levels), such as potatoes and pasta are discouraged. The Sugar Busters Diet adheres to a 30% protein, 40% fat, and 30% carbohydrate meal plan with unlimited portions.

Pros:

꙳ It virtually eliminates most junk foods.

- ∾ It eliminates the excessive "empty" sugar calories that are so prevalent in the modern diet.
- ∾ The food guidelines and meal plans are easy to follow.
- ∾ There is no calorie counting or portion control.

Cons:

- ∾ There is no scientific basis that sugar is toxic.
- ∾ Too many healthy foods are eliminated from the diet.

WEIGHING IN ON LOW-FAT DIETS

How do the traditional low-fat diets stack up against the low-carb diets? Here's a look at one of the most popular of these diets.

The Weight Watchers regimen is the most famous of the high-carbohydrate/low-fat diets. The program was founded by Jean Nidetch in 1967, and began as a food exchange system that limited calories. Dieters could select a certain number of exchanges—or foods selected from each of the major food groups—for each day. It has since become a point system based on the amount of fat, fiber, and calories contained in every food eaten.

The diet establishes a specific number of daily points for each person based on the individual's current weight and desired weight. Dieters have freedom of choice regarding what kind of food is eaten. They're encouraged to write down what foods they eat and their point values in a daily food journal.

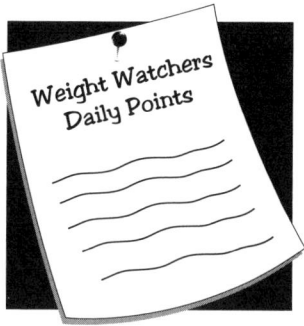

Foods with a high fiber or low fat content have a lower point value on the Weight Watchers plan, and thus can be consumed in greater quantities. A healthy, balanced eating plan low in fat and high in fiber and fruits and vegetables is encouraged.

A new diet plan—offered as an alternative to the point system—was introduced by Weight Watchers in late 2004. It restricts certain foods (foods high in energy density, low in fiber, and refined carbohydrates) but does not require counting points.

The Weight Watchers program offers weekly group meetings, aimed at providing significant emotional support, which is particularly important for individuals with long-term weight reduction goals. A one- to two-pound weekly weight loss is the goal, a rate that is considered the healthiest and easiest to sustain over long periods. The program also encourages paying close attention to what foods are being eaten, and thus can be instrumental in instilling long-term lifestyle changes.

However, it requires a considerable amount of commitment with regard to point-counting, recording one's diet in a journal, and attending weekly meetings. Some people also find the weight loss too slow.

Yet the program is one of the few to be shown effective in producing long-term weight loss. Thus it reduces obesity-related health risks such as heart disease and diabetes. Weight Watchers also has one of the best track records for long-term adherence to healthy eating.

NUTRISYSTEM

This approach to weight loss involves selecting a 28-day program of prepared foods (entrees and snacks) supplemented with fresh grocery items (fruit, vegetables, dairy). The focus is on balanced nutrition and portion control, along with preventing cravings. Online and telephone counseling is available as well. Specific food packages are designed for men, women, and diabetic patients.

REDUCING DISEASE RISK: THE MOST EFFECTIVE DIETS

THE MEDITERRANEAN DIET

Research on the dietary habits of people living near the Mediterranean Sea reveal significantly reduced rates of heart disease and other chronic diseases such as diabetes. More an actual lifestyle than a diet, the Mediterranean plan consists of eating mostly grains, fruits, beans, nuts and vegetables, with little meat, moderate amounts of fish and cheese, and a good deal of olive oil. Garlic is also freely used in the diet. Research indicates that garlic may lower cholesterol, protect against cancer, and also help prevent blood clots. The Mediterranean diet includes drinking moderate amounts of wine, which has been shown to increase HDL,

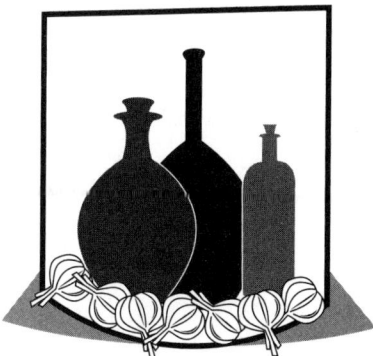

yet can also cause cardiomyopathy, if consumed in excess.

The Mediterranean diet also helps prevent heart disease by removing saturated fats and replacing them with simple, unsaturated fats such as olive oil, which helps regulate cholesterol. The general consensus is the Mediterranean plan provides an ideal healthy diet. The diet requires regular, daily physical activity and can produce weight loss.

Some of the most important contributors to reduced heart disease risk in the Mediterranean diet are the abundant amounts of olive oil and simple unsaturated fatty acids, which are thought to increase HDL (good) cholesterol and lower LDL (bad) cholesterol. Fish, a good source of omega-3 fatty acids, is usually eaten several times a week.

The Mediterranean lifestyle is also slower and more relaxed than ours, which may contribute to its beneficial health effects. The Mediterranean diet and lifestyle is widely recommended by health professionals, and has the added benefit of being easy to follow for vegetarians.

Quick Tips

The Fail-safe Diet: Low in "Energy Density"

Foods with low energy density—containing a lot of water and/or fiber, and low in fat—have less concentrated calories. They'll make you feel more satisfied and less likely to overeat. Thus low energy foods are good choices for those who want to lose weight. A cup and a half of grapes, for instance, is more satisfying than ¼ cup of raisins (both containing 100 calories).

Foods with low energy density include fruits and vegetables and soups—all filling and low in calories. Other good choices include wild and long-grain brown rice, non-sugared hot cereal prepared with water, nonfat or low-fat milk, sugar-free low-fat yogurt and fat-free cottage cheese. Cooked grains have less energy density than breads, so are preferable. Breads with lower energy density include whole wheat tortillas, banana nut and whole wheat breads.

Surprisingly, some foods with the highest energy density (and thus more likely to lead to weight gain) include crackers as well as donuts, pie crust, cheese (even the low-fat variety) and croissants.

Source: *The Volumetrics Weight Control Plan: Feel Full on Fewer Calories.* By Barbara Rolls, Ph.D., and Robert A. Barnett (Harper Collins, 2000)

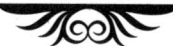

CHAPTER 4

In his popular book, *The Perricone Weight Loss Diet*, Nicholas Perricone, M.D., provides advice on slowing down the aging process and shedding pounds. His diet consists of "anti-inflammatory foods"—low glycemic foods, those rich in omega-3 fatty acids, and brightly colored fruits and vegetables, which are high in antioxidants. He also advises against "pro-inflammatory foods," which cause the body to store fat, increase fatigue and lead to depression. These foods include coffee and sugary and starchy foods, especially those made with sweeteners and flour, according to Dr. Perricone.

Though Dr. Perricone's diet hasn't been scientifically studied, most of its ingredients are healthy—particularly the low glycemic foods, omega-3 fatty acids and antioxidant-rich fruits and vegetables. If followed, the weight loss plan should help one shed pounds successfully.

Though Dr. Perricone's diet hasn't been scientifically studied, most of its ingredients are healthy...

WEIGHT PERFECT

However, the Perricone diet also leans heavily on taking numerous health food supplements, which are both expensive and as yet, unproven.

THE PRITIKIN DIET

This diet was developed in the 1970s by Dr. Nathan Pritikin to help individuals with heart disease. It is a low-fat, high-fiber, low-cholesterol diet and moderate exercise program. Pritikin developed the diet based on his experience in treating his own heart disease.

The Pritikin Diet involves eating restricted amounts of fish and meat, and encourages eating large amounts of whole grains, fruits, and vegetables, and less than 10% of total daily calories from fat. Processed foods such as white pasta and white bread, eggs, and animal fats are eliminated from the diet. Rather than the standard three meals a day, it encourages eating six or seven meals a day, and portions are unrestricted as long as the foods meet the program's criteria. The diet has come under criticism for being too stringent, and not allowing "healthy" fats.

The more recent revised Pritikin Lifetime Eating Plan, established by Dr. Pritikin's son,

Robert, includes healthy omega-3 fatty acids such as those found in salmon, and some oils, but only in limited amounts.

THE ORNISH DIET

Dr. Dean Ornish developed a diet similar to the Pritikin diet. It emphasizes low-fat, high-fiber foods that are filling but low in calories. It is primarily plant-based and excludes all animal products and nuts and seeds. The only oils permitted are canola oil and oils with omega-3 fatty acids. Caffeine is prohibited, but small amounts of alcohol, sugar, and salt are permitted. It promotes heart health and provides anti-cancer benefits since it contains no cholesterol, is low is saturated fats, and high in antioxidants and fiber. The diet exists in two forms: the Reversal Diet, for people with known heart disease; and the Prevention Diet, for people who do not have heart disease but do have cholesterol levels of 150 or higher.

Both the Pritikin and Ornish diets have been criticized for being too low in fat and for not including enough essential fatty acids. There is some controversy as to whether the amount of fat allowed in these diets is sufficient for the absorption of certain vitamins (A, D, E, and K) and for a healthy diet in general. However both diets can produce significant weight loss. They've also been shown by scientific studies to reverse atherosclerosis, and to decrease risk of cardiovascular disease.

THE DANGERS OF YO-YO DIETING

Research on the dangers of yo-yo dieting—losing and gaining weight repeatedly—has been contradictory. However, some studies do show that yo-yo dieting (also called weight cycling) can be associated with ill health effects. A study of 2,476 nurses in the *International Journal of Obesity and Related Metabolic Disorders* in September 2004, for instance, showed that those women who practiced yo-yo dieting were less likely to maintain weight loss. They were more likely to regain weight after dieting, less likely to exercise and were at greater risk for binge eating and bulimia.

...those women who practiced yo-yo dieting were less likely to maintain weight loss.

Some studies have suggested that weight cycling may be associated with high blood pressure, high cholesterol and gallbladder disease, though much of this evidence is not conclusive. Contrary to myth, however, weight cycling does not affect metabolism or the amount of fat tissue around the abdomen.

A study published in the *Journal of the American Dietetic Association* reveals that frequent intentional weight loss may be linked to a decrease in the body's levels of NK (natural killer) cells and lowered immune function.

NK cells are an important part of the body's immune system. They protect against viral infections and microbial pathogens. Low levels of NK cells have also been linked to a higher risk of cancer.

The study evaluated the weight loss habits of 114 healthy, overweight, sedentary postmenopausal women. Women who intentionally lost 10 pounds or more over the last 20 years had lower NK cytotoxicity levels than those who did not intentionally lose weight. Frequent intentional weight loss or weight cycling was also associated with a decrease in the number of NK cells.

Should You Really Diet?

In women with high BMIs, lifestyle changes may be more effective in promoting good health than continued dieting, according to a study published in the *Journal of the American Dietetic Association* in June, 2004. In the study, the researchers found that many obese women had made repeated attempts at weight loss through dieting—a strategy that eventually undermined their health, increased their tendency to gain weight and led to feelings of low self-esteem.

The study collected self-reported dieting histories of 149 women with high body mass index (BMI) between 30 and 77. Many women in the study said frequent dieting "undermined their health and self-esteem" and contributed to weight gain throughout their lives. The feelings these women now attach to dieting—and the unintended negative health consequences of repeated dieting—suggest that different treatment goals for the obese are needed.

Initially, the women interviewed in the study often felt satisfied and empowered after losing weight. However, after they failed to maintain weight loss or gained more weight, they often felt feelings of shame, body hatred, humiliation, and deprivation.

Some of their comments were compelling:

> *"As a child, every doctor visit was a lecture about how fat I was and how there needed to be something done about it."*

> *"Amphetamines (I used to lose weight) made me so jittery that I pulled all my hair out of the top of my head. I have never been a big eater and weight came back on immediately plus more. I felt such shame."*

Due to their lack of success with dieting in the past, these and many other obese people may required altered strategies of weight management. Dietitians and other clinicians need to acknowledge and respect the negative feelings that their clients may have about dieting. Rather than recommending a weight loss diet, clinicians should advise lifestyle changes that improve metabolic health and reduce risk of chronic disabilities.

The lowest number of NK cells, in fact, was found in women who reported the highest number of weight loss episodes.

However, those who maintained their weight loss for the longest periods of time were more likely to have greater numbers of NK cells and stronger immune function. Previously published studies (Nieman et al, 1998, Scanga et al, 1998) reveal that exercise may minimize the negative effects of frequent intentional weight loss on immune response. Exercise, combined with healthy lifestyle and dietary changes, can also prevent weight cycling.

The researchers concluded that yo-yo dieting may have long-term effects on immune function, especially among those who are sedentary or who fail to maintain weight loss.

THE BOTTOM LINE

Research is providing new data daily regarding how our bodies process food, and how and why we gain weight. Many fad diets do provide short-term results, and some are supported by scientific research. But the success of fad diets lies not in choosing foods from particular food groups, but because—like all diets—they limit calorie intake. And too many calories is the primary cause of weight gain. Following a diet program—any diet— also forces people to pay attention to what they eat, often resulting in healthier food choices. Most people, however, who follow fad diets usually gain back the weight they have lost.

The view supported by the National Institutes of Health (NIH), the American Heart Association, the Centers for Disease Control (CDC), and numerous other organizations is that the way to achieve and maintain a healthy weight is to eat sensible amounts of healthy foods. Reducing calories is what counts, along with eating a nutritious, healthy diet high in fiber and rich in fruits and vegetables, with a moderate amount of healthy fats.

To quote Dean Ornish: "To the degree you move in a healthful direction on the food spectrum, you're likely to feel better, lose weight, and gain health."

CHAPTER 4

Chapter 5

emotions & overeating:
how to stop the cycle

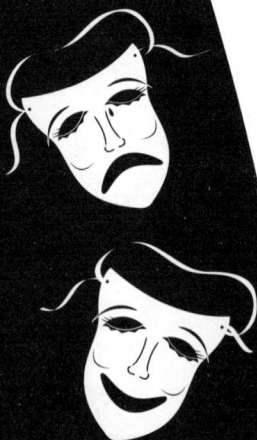

"Life itself is the proper binge."
~ *Julia Child*

Almost everyone acknowledges the connection between emotions and eating. Happiness at an unexpected raise, panic when the stock market plummets 600 points, stress when the kids are sick and you're trying to meet a deadline at work—all can trigger unplanned eating.

The relationship between emotions and eating is complex. Why do some people respond to emotions by eating, others by drinking or smoking, and still others by exercising or talking with a trusted friend? Why do some people gain weight when they're depressed and others lose weight? Scientists have been wrestling with these and other questions for many years.

There is a complicated but fascinating relationship between what we feel, what we eat, and what we weigh. And there are strategies for gaining awareness and control over emotional eating.

Probably the earliest study of emotions and eating was conducted during World War II at the University of Minnesota by nutritionist Ancel Keys. He was charged with developing a nutritious, portable, and stable diet for men in battle (he was the inventor of the "K ration"). In the course of his research, he fed volunteers a diet consisting of approximately half their normal caloric intake in order to study the effects of semi-starvation. As they lost weight, the men became increasingly irritable, depressed, argumentative, and unmotivated, and he found that these emotional problems only subsided once the study ended and they had regained the weight they had lost.

Hilde Bruch, a psychoanalyst in the Freudian tradition, believed that overeating and overweight were the result of powerful unmet needs for affection and nurturing. As food and nurturing are intimately entwined from earliest infancy, she proposed that an affection-starved individual would use food as a substitute for human contact to satisfy his or her need for affection. Bruch was one

...overeating and overweight were the result of powerful unmet needs for affection and nurturing.

of the first to suggest that obesity was a symptom of an underlying emotional illness.

In the 1970s, psychologists Janet Polivy and Peter Herman developed a novel theory about the relationship between emotions, eating, and weight. They proposed that there were two styles of eating: restrained and unrestrained. Restrained eating is typical of frequent dieters. It means constantly resisting desired foods, and worrying about food and eating. Unrestrained eating is typical of non-dieters who eat what they like without worrying about health or weight.

Numerous studies revealed that those who score high on restraint respond more emotionally to life events, and worry more about losing control over eating. Polivy and Herman believed that this increased emotional response was a result of dieting, not of being overweight or obese. Since dieting can heighten emotions, frequent dieters risk experiencing feelings that are powerful enough to cause them to overeat.

These theories have been influential in shaping current thinking about emotions, eating, weight, and dieting. It is now widely accepted, for instance, that overweight and obese individuals are not emotionally ill. In fact, the *Diagnostic and Statistical Manual Fifth Edition* (DSM-5), does not list overweight or obesity as psychiatric disorders. But the work of Keys, Stunkard, Polivy and Herman, and good old common sense tell us that what we eat, and by extension what we weigh, is influenced by what we feel.

THE POWER OF EMOTIONS

Perhaps the most influential theory about emotions—and how they can powerfully influence our lives—was developed by psychologist Richard Lazarus. Lazarus believed that strong emotions engage us completely—our thoughts, our needs and desires, and even our bodies. Strong emotional reactions often reveal that an important goal or value is being advanced or placed at risk.

Indeed, emotions have both a mental and a physical component. When we're angry, for instance, we may have thoughts of revenge (mental), and experience muscle tension (physical). When frightened, we may feel a "knot in our stomach" (physical) and have a disturbing sense that something bad is about to happen (mental). The breakup of a relationship causes anger and sadness, as well as tension, increased heart rate, and increased blood pressure. Different emotions bring about different mental and physical sensations. According to Lazarus, emotions almost always originate from an interaction with another person.

Emotions have both a mental and a physical component.

DEPRESSION: DOES IT CAUSE OVEREATING?

The word "depression" is used in many ways. Someone who feels "sad", "down", or "blue" for a few hours or days may say they are "depressed." But true depression is an illness, an extreme form of sadness or the blues. When sadness or the blues lasts for a prolonged period and significantly interferes with daily life, it crosses over into clinical depression.

Clinical depression is considered a "mood disorder." Often called the "common cold" of mental illness, it affects one out of every ten people at some time during their lives. Women are affected twice as often as men.

Clinical or major depression can affect eating habits in several ways. It can cause severe loss of appetite and great difficulty eating anything at all, or increased appetite and cravings for certain foods, such as carbohydrates. The first type of depression leads to weight loss and the second to weight gain. Adults who suffer from major depression as adolescents tend to weigh more as adults than those who did not have depression as teenagers.

Not surprisingly, binge eaters have also been found to be more depressed than people who do not binge eat, regardless of weight.

Yet the relationship between depression and weight is actually quite complex. Several studies have shown that depression can sometimes result *from* dieting, especially with very rapid weight loss.

The relationship between depression and weight is actually quite complex. Psychiatrist Albert Stunkard of the University of Pennsylvania theorized that dieting results in emotional disturbance. He evaluated the effects of dieting on 25 young women, and discovered that approximately one third of them experienced first anxiety and then depression during and after weight loss. A follow-up study revealed that half the women reported they felt nervous, weak, and irritable during a previous dieting attempt.

Dieting can be taxing, requiring considerable attention to the purchase, preparation, and consumption of each and every item of food. And given the difficulty of sticking with a diet, the transgressions that occur for most people can lead to feeling angry, despondent, and inadequate. So, while there is evidence that depression and overweight are related, it is not clear which is cause and which is effect.

There is even some evidence that depression appears to cause unhealthy fat deposits in

CHAPTER 5

particular areas of the body. Known as "visceral fat," it deposits itself around internal organs, such as the heart and liver and deep inside the abdomen—the fat that creates the so-called "apple shape." Visceral fat—as opposed to "surface fat" that is deposited just under the skin—has been linked to higher risk of hypertension, heart disease, stroke, diabetes and some forms of cancer. High levels of the hormone cortisol may play a role in the development of visceral fat.

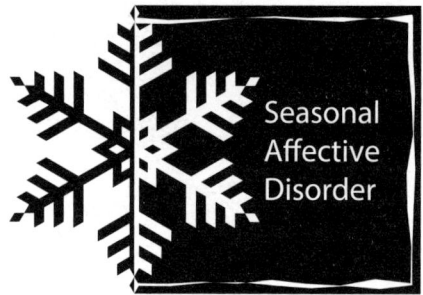

"Seasonal affective disorder" or SAD, can also affect weight gain. SAD occurs during winter months in more northern climates, and the reduced number of daylight hours is the main culprit. As with other depressions, SAD sufferers frequently crave carbohydrates and gain weight during the winter.

But there is good news: Depression is treatable, and many of the treatments that elevate mood can also help normalize eating habits and facilitate weight loss. If you experience sadness that continues for more than a few weeks, or if you feel so unhappy or exhausted that you can't get through your day or you can't get a whole night's sleep, see your physician. Numerous medications can improve how you feel and function in several weeks, especially when accompanied by counseling and improved sleep.

If, on the other hand, you feel down for only a few days or a couple of weeks, then the following strategies may help you both feel better and eat better:

How to Improve Your Mood

Get moving. If you're down or mildly depressed, you may feel lethargic. The very thought of getting out of bed may seem like a huge obstacle. But if you can coax yourself to move—even for just a few minutes—your mood may improve. Research consistently finds that even a little exercise elevates mood. And since physical activity burns calories and helps regulate the hormones and neurochemicals that increase appetite, it can also check cravings. And reduced cravings help keep your weight control efforts on track.

CHAPTER 5

Remember that a *little* activity beats *no* activity. So, if you can only motivate yourself to walk around the block, it's a start! Try breaking down physical activity into small units. Three ten-minute walks add up to thirty minutes of exercise, and will boost your mood and decrease appetite.

Remember that a little activity beats no activity.

Do something you like. Feelings of sadness and even clinical depression can signal *too little fun* in your life. The solution? Do *something pleasurable* every day. It doesn't have to involve a lot of expense or planning; it just has to be something you enjoy doing. Taking a bubble bath with scented oil and candles, calling a friend, or listening to some favorite music may improve your mood and distract you from food at the same time.

Start a Mood/Food Journal. Research shows that keeping track of what you feel and eat can improve your mood and eating patterns. Buy a small notebook just for this purpose, and write down any powerful emotions you feel and the foods you eat as a result. Keep the journal for at least three weeks and then review it for patterns. What emotions pop up repeatedly? What foods do you eat when they occur? As you begin to see the connection between your emotions and your eating patterns, you may start to gain control over both.

Modify your diet. Depression and excessive consumption of sugar and/or caffeine don't mix. Dietitian Elizabeth Somer writing in her book, *Food and Mood* (Henry Holt & Co., 1999) suggests avoiding all foods containing sugar and caffeine for three weeks and then re-evaluating your mood. She also suggests that your mood will improve if you:

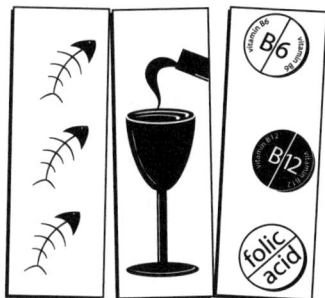

∾ Eat fish at least three times a week

∾ Avoid alcohol or drink in moderation

∾ Make sure you are getting enough vitamins B_6, B_{12} and folic acid

That was good advice in 1999. It's good advice now.

CHAPTER 5

Anger is one of our most common emotions. And anger and eating are closely linked. Anger makes us want to take action against a person or situation, and it has been found that *binge eating* is often used to cope with anger.

Binge-eating, in which large amounts of food are consumed rapidly and usually in secret, is fairly prevalent. It is estimated that 6% of the general population, including people of all weights, and 30% of weight loss program participants are binge eaters. A study published in 2003 in the *Journal of Psychosomatic Research* found a direct relation between anger and the impulse to binge among obese individuals.

Anger can be expressed directly or indirectly, or suppressed. Strong physical sensations accompany anger, including sensations of "simmering", "stewing", and "festering". Anger can build up and be released in explosive outbursts or in indirect "passive-aggressive" behavior like sarcasm and nagging. Recent studies have found that, like depression, anger can affect where fat is deposited on the body. The most dangerous form of fat,

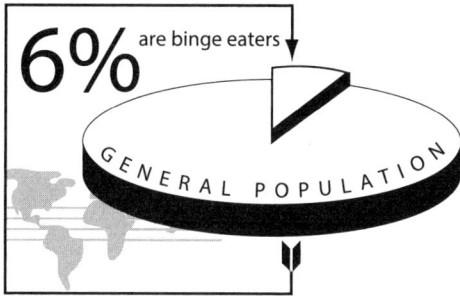

6% are binge eaters

GENERAL POPULATION

surrounding internal organs (visceral fat), tends to be more common among those who feel angry a lot, express their anger outwardly, and have generally hostile attitudes. Patients with chronic anger may also experience chronic pain and inadequate sleep.

CALMING ANGER

If you find yourself frequently angry, or if your journal shows that you eat when you are angry, the anger management strategies below may be useful:

Turn the tables. Ask yourself what's eating you. If you suspect that anger plays a role in your binge eating, ask yourself what is bothering you when you reach for food. Just seeing the connection is the first step to finding non-food ways to reduce your anger.

Assert yourself. You may find yourself alternating between "stuffing" your feelings (and your mouth), and exploding uncontrollably. Neither reaction is satisfying, and both can lead to frustration, guilt, and unwanted pounds. Instead, try walking the middle ground: assert yourself. Assertion is different from aggression in that you say what you feel and want calmly and strongly, not nastily. It differs from passivity in that you speak directly to the person you are angry at, make eye contact, and do not skirt the issue.

...ask yourself what is bothering you when you reach for food.

An example of three ways to handle a potentially anger-causing situation. **Situation:** For the third time this week, a friend asks if you can drive her son home from school. You say:

- ∞ **Aggressive:** *I'm sick and tired of you asking me to drive your son home. Don't you think I have other things to do with my time?*
- ∞ **Passive-aggressive:** *Well, I guess so. I have to make a birthday dinner tonight, but I suppose I can drive him home.*
- ∞ **Assertive:** *I'm really sorry. I'd like to help you out if I could. But today just isn't going to work for me.*

Release your anger physically. Anger is a powerful emotion. A far better response than "stuffing" anger is to express it—constructively. Physical activity can release the build-up of adrenaline and other chemicals that accumulate in the body when you're angry. Walk around the block a few times, take a bike ride, or swim some laps at a local pool. These alternatives will leave you feeling more relaxed and less worked up.

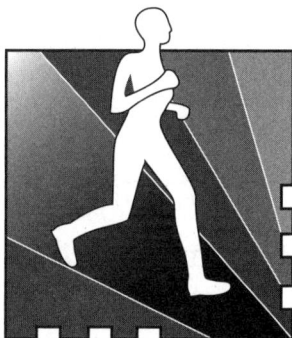

EATING DISORDERS: HIDDEN EMOTIONS

Anorexia nervosa is an eating disorder in which an individual, usually an adolescent or young adult, stops eating and, may die from the resulting malnutrition if not treated. Many experts believe unconscious anger plays a significant role in the development of this disorder:

Generally the "good child", the anorexic adolescent or young adult feels little control over the important issues in her life, and refusing to eat becomes the only way of exerting power and independence from the family. For this reason, family therapy is often considered important in treating anorexia, along with cognitive-behavioral therapy and nutrition counseling. The goal of family sessions is to help the parents accept and support their child's increasing independence and need for autonomy.

Bulimia nervosa, typically called bulimia, is another eating disorder. Someone with bulimia eats a lot of food in a short amount of time (called bingeing) and then tries to prevent weight gain by purging. Purging is done in these ways:

∾ making oneself vomit

∾ taking laxatives

Bulimia nervosa is often a way in which people attempt to feel more in control of their lives, and ease stress and anxiety. There is no single cause of bulimia, but genetics, stressful events or life changes and the pressure in our culture to be thin may all play a role.

Research shows that people with bulimia may have low self-esteem, experience feelings of helplessness, and dislike the way they look. In families where there is a great deal of emphasis on appearance and diet, children are more likely to develop bulimia.

ANXIETY & STRESS

Anxiety has long been considered an eating trigger.

Anxiety is defined as a complex feeling of apprehension, fear, and worry, often accompanied by pulmonary, cardiac, and other physical sensations. Chronic anxiety takes its toll on the body, elevating one's risk of chronic disease. Anxiety has long been considered an eating trigger.

Some studies suggest that if you are aware of why you are anxious, and you feel you have some control over the situation, you are less likely to eat in response. Anxiety that you can't put your finger on may be more likely to provoke eating.

Stress is your reaction to something you consider a challenge or a threat.

While stressors can be serious, such as a job loss, a death in the family or of a friend, or a divorce, some researchers believe it is the everyday annoyances which, taken together, can overwhelm us.

CHAPTER 5

When a stressful event occurs, the adrenal glands produce hormones called "glucocorticoids." As increasing amounts of glucocorticoids course through the body, they counteract the body's stress response and help restore calm. But when stress is frequent and repetitive, the glucocorticoids begin to function differently. Instead of restoring calm, they actually maintain the state of stress. The result is often overeating and deposition of visceral fat.

With chronic stress from daily hassles, the brain—and therefore the body—remains on high alert. As high levels of stress hormones continually surge through the body, they cause physical, emotional, and behavioral problems that many people cope with by turning to food.

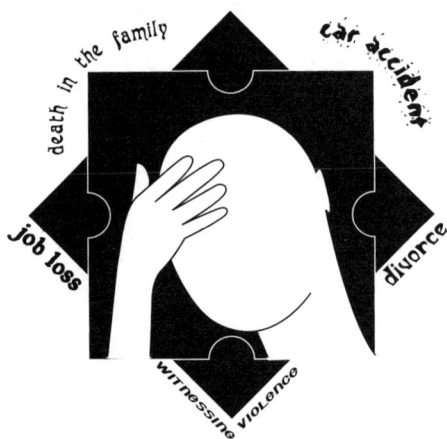

STOPPING THE STRESS-EATING CYCLE

If anxiety and stress are among the triggers that lead you to overeat, try some of these strategies :

- *Be intentionally active.* Go on a walk or a bike ride, clean out a closet, do some cleaning or yard work. Change your mental state.

- *Look to friends for support.* If you think stress is causing you to overeat, try talking to a friend instead.

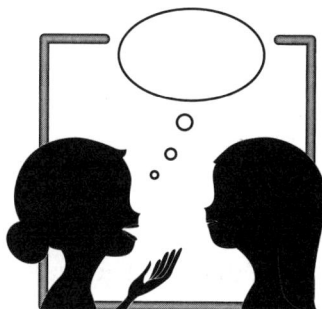

- *Don't buy junk foods.* Avoid having a lot of high-fat, high-sugar foods in your house. Don't go grocery shopping when you're feeling stressed—so you won't buy unhealthy foods on impulse.

- *Try some healthy snacks.* For snacks, try low-fat, low-calorie food, such as fresh fruit, unbuttered popcorn, or whole grain cereal.

- *Eat a nutritious diet.* If you're not eating a balanced diet, you're more likely to fall prey to emotional eating. Eat five to six small meals per day to make sure you feel satisfied, and your energy doesn't flag. In that way, you're less likely to reach for an unhealthy pick-me-up snack.

- Turn your attention to *prayer, meditation, volunteer work,* or *creative efforts.*

MEDITATION:
LEARN THE RELAXATION RESPONSE

WHAT IS MEDITATION?

Meditation is a way to quiet the mind and relax the body It is a way of becoming more awake, more relaxed and more deliberate about what you are doing. It is easy to learn but somewhat difficult to perfect, and has many documented physiologic and psychological benefits.

Herbert Benson, M.D., a cardiologist at Harvard University, was one of the first scientists to show that meditation

Meditating twice a day for 20 minutes each time is ideal...

has beneficial health effects. He has found in a series of scientific studies that meditation can reduce hypertension, anxiety and depression, for example. The goal of meditation is to achieve what Dr. Benson terms "the relaxation response." In this state, there is a decrease in heart rate, metabolism and respiratory rate, as well as a reduction of stress. (*Beyond the Relaxation Response.* Berkeley Books, 1985)

While there are numerous ways to meditate, one straightforward method has been developed by Dr. Benson. His suggested meditation involves finding a 20-minute time period when you are unlikely to be interrupted, putting on comfortable clothing, and sitting in a quiet, comfortable place.

The Benson Meditation

ॐ Either close your eyes, or choose a focal point across the room. Take one or two deep breaths, inhaling through the mouth, and exhaling through the nose.

ॐ Now, select a word to repeat silently to yourself. The word you choose can be anything, but it is helpful if the word suggests something peaceful, calming or pleasant. "Peace," "calm," or "one" are some examples. Some people also use a spiritual phrase that has special meaning for them.

ॐ Repeat your chosen word or "mantra" silently for 20 minutes. Keep in mind that exact timing isn't necessary, so there's no need to watch the clock. As you meditate, thoughts and sensations from inside you and distractions from outside will creep into your consciousness. When you find yourself thinking about something other than your word, very gently bring yourself back to it. Don't be harsh on yourself—distractions are to be expected, especially early on. So, when you find your mind wandering, just re-focus.

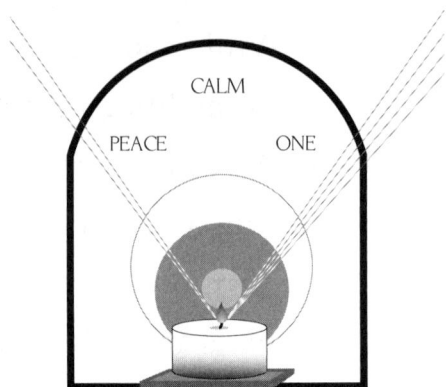

ɷ After about 20 minutes, slowly and gently bring yourself back to reality. Meditating twice a day for 20 minutes each time is ideal, but once a day for 20 minutes is helpful, too. If you decide to meditate, give it at least three months and then evaluate how well it is working. You may find yourself, like many others, impressed by the benefits it produces.

DEFEATING EMOTIONAL EATING

One approach to handling emotional eating was developed at Duke University—and adapted from behavioral coping strategies created by the self-help program Alcoholics Anonymous. When you are tempted to eat, ask yourself if you are: *H*ungry, *A*ngry, *L*onely, or *T*ired (the mnemonic **"H-A-L-T"**). If you are hungry (you haven't eaten for several hours and your stomach is growling), sit down to a meal or eat a healthy snack. If you are angry, lonely, tired, or even bored, try one of the suggestions below:

Plan ahead. Well before the urge to eat strikes, plan alternative ways of handling your emotions. If boredom is a trigger, get involved in a new activity to add variety and increase your self-esteem. If you are lonely, plan ahead to see a friend or join with friends in an activity you enjoy. If you are tired, try eating a nutritious breakfast to boost your energy, or take a 20-minute "power nap." Meditation and physical activity can also help reduce feelings of fatigue.

Replace negative thoughts with positive ones. For example, if you tell yourself "my parents were overweight, I'm doomed to be fat," try replacing it with "my genes may predispose me to overweight, but they can't make me overeat."

Talk to a trusted friend. Everyone needs at least one confidante. If you can speak candidly about what is bothering you to even one other person, chances are you'll feel better without overeating.

OVER-EATING: TOO MUCH OF A GOOD THING?

Negative emotions aren't the only ones that can lead us to make unwise food choices. Celebrations are also linked with the tendency to overindulge. Joyful occasions and festivities often center around food—and often tempt us with lots of available high calorie, high fat food.

Obviously, it is desirable to feel positive and joyful, and to have many happy occasions in life. Try some of the tips below to help keep your good times from sabotaging your weight control efforts:

CELEBRATING WITHOUT GAINING

∾ If you have a special occasion meal coming up, eat lighter for a couple of days before. You will feel much freer to indulge if you have made room for a celebratory meal.

∾ Start your celebration with a green salad: A salad is not only chock full of vitamins, but it can take the edge off your appetite and make it easier to control what you eat. Watch out for

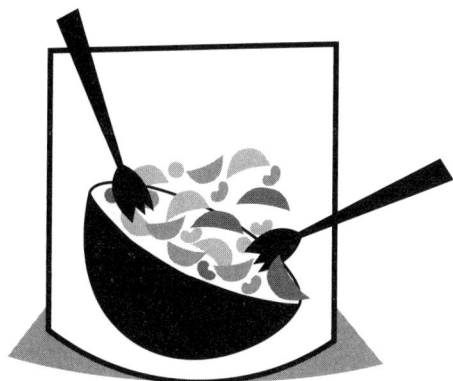

fattening salad dressings. Alternatively, try eating some yogurt or a snack of fruit and nuts before the party.

∾ Get yourself moving: When you feel good, it is easier to move. Take advantage of this extra energy by going for a walk or engaging in a physical activity you enjoy. It will add to your celebratory mood, as well as cutting your appetite.

TREATING EMOTIONAL EATING

PSYCHOLOGICAL COUNSELING

If despite your best efforts, you find yourself eating to cope with intense feelings, psychological counseling can help. Most therapists use some form of cognitive-behavioral therapy to help people with emotional weight problems. Cognitive-behavioral therapy is a fairly short-term treatment, usually lasting a few months to a year. It helps people discover their personal emotional triggers and develop new behaviors

CHAPTER 5

that can cut their dependence on food. If emotions continually sabotage your dieting efforts, psychological counseling may help.

Cognitive-behavioral therapy is a fairly short-term treatment...

In cognitive behavioral therapy, you will learn to reduce stress and replace negative thoughts about yourself, your body, and your life, with positive ones. For example, one client who defined herself as a "coping eater," had a hyperactive son she couldn't control, a demanding husband she couldn't please, and days full of stressful work. Her negative feelings about her inability to cope were always compounded by the guilt she felt when she overate. Her therapist first helped her let go of the belief that she was a helpless victim of circumstances. Then, he helped her begin to satisfy her needs without overeating—by becoming more assertive.

They confronted her ambivalence about losing weight, and then looked for new ways of satisfying the emotional needs previously met by food. These strategies included asking her husband to join her in marriage counseling and then, to bolster her self-esteem and lessen her boredom, enrolling in a course at her local community college. By brainstorming with her therapist, she was able to draw up a list of non-eating activities to deal with intense emotions: calling a friend, taking a hot bath, or walking around the neighborhood.

In addition to developing specific behavioral alternatives to eating, psychological counseling can help you figure out what is bothering you and take steps to change disturbing situations. Even if you can't change a situation, counseling can help you change how you think about it and, as a result, how you feel about it.

Binge eaters also respond well to cognitive behavioral therapy, especially when they work with treatment teams, including psychotherapists, physicians, nutritionists, and nurses.

Support Groups

Finding a supportive group of people who share your problems can help you get through the feelings that are leading you to overeat. Many people find that programs such as Weight Watchers or TOPS (Take Off Pounds Sensibly) provide the support they need.

CHAPTER 5

In general, there are two simple rules for gaining control over your life:

- ∾ If a stressful situation can be changed, find a way to change it.
- ∾ If a stressful situation can't be changed, find the best way to live with it.

These are the principles of the "Serenity Prayer" which asks for the "courage to change what can be changed, the serenity to accept what can't be changed, and the wisdom to know the difference."

THE BOTTOM LINE

An increasing amount of research now shows that our emotions are often linked to our eating behaviors. Overeating is a coping strategy—and an understandable one—that many of us use to deal with intense emotions and troublesome problems. Unfortunately, once the food is gone, the problems often remain.

Instead try developing new ways of dealing with life's frustrations. Choose other ways to reduce stress—exercise, relaxation techniques, finding a supportive friend—that don't depend

WEIGHT PERFECT

on overeating. And begin to think positively about your ability to effect change in your life.

Forgiving yourself and others is important too. Everyone slips up and overeats occasionally. Just know that every day is a new opportunity to eat and live more healthfully.

Chapter 6
controlling cravings

"There is a charm about the forbidden that
makes it unspeakably desirable."

∾ Mark Twain

"Inside some of us is a thin person
struggling to get out, but they can usually
be sedated with a few pieces of chocolate
cake."

∾ Author Unknown

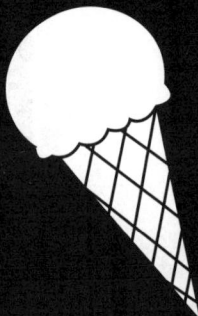

Food cravings occur in almost everyone, but unfortunately, they can play havoc with health. Like the sirens of Greek mythology, food cravings can feel tempting—almost irresistible.

The catch is that food cravings are most likely to occur when you're on a diet, and trying to restrict your intake of certain foods, often your favorite foods.

The good news is that food cravings do not have to control your life or your diet. It is possible to moderate food cravings—and even give in to them occasionally—without sacrificing your weight loss efforts. In this chapter, we'll give you some tips on how to keep food cravings from sabotaging healthy eating.

THE PROBLEM WITH FOOD CRAVINGS

Have you ever found yourself driving along, your thoughts drifting fondly in the direction of a hot fudge sundae? The rich ice cream, dense with vanilla beans, and thick dark fudge seems to call your name.

What you're experiencing is a food craving, defined as "an intense desire or longing" for a particular food.

What's the difference between a food craving and hunger? Hunger produces physical sensations, such as a growling stomach, lightheadedness, and weakness, all caused by the body's need for fuel. Hunger can be satisfied by many different foods, but a craving can be satisfied only with a specific food—usually a soothing, sweet or fat-laden food, such as chocolate or French fries.

Food cravings are especially common among women. Almost 100% of young adult women and almost 70% of men report having had at least one food craving during the past year. Eighty-five percent of people who

Food cravings are especially common among women.

experience cravings say they give in to them a least half the time.

Consider the story of Alexa. As a freshman at college, she found herself enjoying life with her new friends, as well as her newfound freedom. Every night around 10 p.m., Alexa and her friends would order pizza, replete with sausage, pepperoni, and salami, from their local pizza parlor.

After a few weeks of indulging in late-night pizza snacks, however, Alexa found that it was becoming more difficult to zip up her favorite jeans. Could those late night pizza parties be the reason? While she considered passing up the pizza, the luscious cheesy aroma seduced Alexa night after night. Before she knew it, Alexa was downing two slices and a couple of glasses of sugary soda every night—and she soon had 10 extra pounds to show for it.

As Alexa discovered, the problem with food cravings is that they can lead to weight gain. Most people tend to crave calorie rich foods, usually loaded with fat or sugar. But food cravings do not have to derail your diet. You can give in to an occasional craving and still lose or maintain your weight.

THE FOODS WE CRAVE

One of the most interesting facts about cravings is that they tend to be quite individual. Most people crave foods high in both carbohydrates and fat. One example is pizza—high in carbohydrates (bread dough) as well as fat (cheese and oil). But while your favorite carb craving may be double cheese pizza, your best friend's favorite food may be chocolate chip brownies. People who experience carbohydrate cravings can have a desire for savory foods such as pasta, pizza or chips, or for sweet foods, such as chocolate, ice cream, cookies, and cake.

Surprisingly, people can also experience cravings for protein-rich foods—usually foods high in both protein and fat, such as steak, cheese, or even milk.

Another common craving is for "comfort foods" usually those associated with positive childhood experiences. Dishes that were commonly served at family celebrations or traditional holiday meals such as Thanksgiving and Christmas dinners often

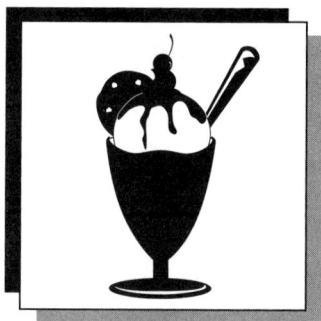

become linked with positive memories. That's why foods such as mashed potatoes, green bean casserole and stuffing can arouse general feelings of comfort and relaxation. Comfort foods can be carbohydrates or proteins, and can fall into the sweet or savory category.

What causes food cravings? Research tells us that the cause of our food cravings resides in the brain's pleasure centers.

In 2004, scientists at the US Department of Energy's Brookhaven National Laboratory found that brain metabolism increases 24% or more when food stimuli are presented to a hungry person. Just being close to a tempting food, smelling it, and tasting it on the tongue (without swallowing it) excites the brain and increases brain metabolism. A section of the brain that influences motivation and pleasure, called the right orbitofrontal cortex, is particularly sensitive to both hunger and the desire for food.

Research has found that cocaine cravings are also associated with the right orbitofrontal cortex, providing evidence that food cravings and drug addiction share a common brain pathway.

Some scientists theorize that the brain centers stimulated by opiates such as heroin are also stimulated by craved foods. Studies are currently underway examining how cravings are affected when opiate receptors in the brain are blocked. The next generation of weight loss medications may well rely upon this very mechanism.

The question remains: Can certain foods be as addictive as drugs? Although evidence does indicate a link between food and narcotic addiction, it is far from conclusive. Scientists do know that people abstaining from drugs, alcohol, and nicotine develop cravings for carbohydrates, for instance. When drugs such as naloxone, which blocks the effects of opiates, are administered, people report reduced cravings for nicotine, alcohol, and drugs. Naloxone also reduces food intake in normal volunteers, and can make sweet foods less appealing.

Have you ever found yourself reaching for a chocolate bar or sugary doughnut when a deadline is looming, or when you're feeling depressed and overwhelmed by life's stresses?

Scientific studies do suggest that people crave carbohydrate-rich foods as a way of self-treating depression or negative mood states. It is well accepted that carbohydrate-laden foods increase levels of the amino acid tryptophan. Once it reaches the brain, tryptophan increases synthesis of serotonin, a

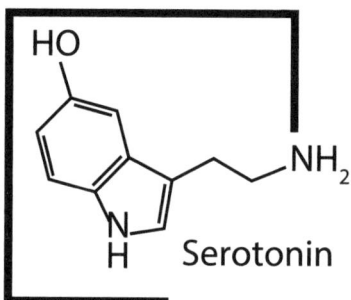

HO

NH$_2$

N
H   Serotonin

critical mood regulator. Serotonin increases feelings of well being and relaxation.

Some scientific evidence indicates that carbohydrate-rich foods elevate mood, according to studies published by Judith Wurtman, Ph.D. As a result, people begin to associate carbohydrate-laden foods with feeling better, and start to desire these foods whenever they feel down.

DIETING:
DOES IT CAUSE FOOD CRAVINGS?

It's ironic, but dieting can lead to food cravings. Most diets restrict food intake in many ways, and most of these restrictions lead to food cravings—especially in the first few weeks. The Atkins diet, for example, severely restricts carbohydrates and Weight Watchers and diets promoted by the U.S. government encourage restriction of fats and calories.

The more restrictive the diet, the more likely you are to experience food cravings. Atkins dieters enjoying a hearty breakfast of eggs and bacon may long to add a slice of toast with jam, or home-fried potatoes, to their meal. On conventional diets, high carbohydrate and high fat foods are often very limited, and dieters often crave these foods.

When following the Sugar Busters diet, which advocates eliminating all refined sugars, withdrawal symptoms can develop, including headache, dizziness or lightheadedness. But these symptoms tend to resolve after a few weeks, as do sugar cravings.

During the Biosphere project, in which volunteers lived in a self-contained community designed to provide all of life's needs, volunteers' diets consisted primarily of grains and vegetables they grew themselves. After about a year, the volunteers found themselves craving chocolate, cheese, and other fatty foods that were not available within the Biosphere.

A common diet strategy is to severely restrict or eliminate certain foods, such as sugar and/or other simple carbohydrates, such as breads, to keep cravings under control. But extreme dietary restraint can lead to binge eating. Some experts believe that deciding whether or not to severely restrict foods on a diet should depend on the amount of self-control an individual has. Some people may only need a miniature chocolate candy or two to satisfy a craving, and can still stick to their diet. Then there are those of us who start out eating one or two candies, and end up polishing off a whole bag of chocolates. So for

A common diet strategy is to severely restrict or eliminate certain foods...

these dieters, eliminating those first few pieces of candy might be the best choice.

LATE-NIGHT CRAVINGS

People who skip breakfast or other meals, or snack frequently on sugary foods throughout the day often report late-night carbohydrate and fat cravings. One strategy to defeat late night cravings is to regularly have breakfast. Those who eat breakfast daily are less likely to experience frequent late-night cravings.

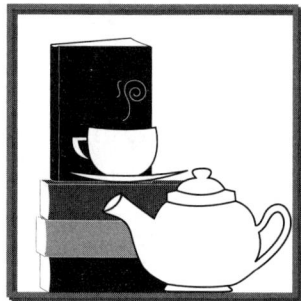

Late-night cravings appear to be a conditioned response. Like Pavlov's dogs, people come to associate certain times of day (such as late evening), and typical activities (such as watching television) with eating. These surrounding conditions are what psychologists call "cues." However, if you change the "cues" you can overcome your typical late night cravings. For instance, make it a habit to read a book and drink chamomile tea—instead of watching TV and chowing down on buttered popcorn each evening.

Curbing Cravings: What can you do?

The tips below may help keep your craving from spiraling out of control:

- *When you feel a craving coming on, do something besides eating.* Go for a walk, type an e-mail, drink a glass of water, or decide to go to yoga class. You may then be able to reduce the intensity of the craving, or eliminate it altogether.

- *Find a food that has the characteristics you crave but with less fat and/or sugar.* Raw broccoli never fulfilled anyone's craving for chocolate cake or cookies. But a frozen fat-free chocolate fudge bar just might. If you want a cookie, try lower-fat, lower-calorie varieties, such as graham cracker, ginger snap, or Fig Newton. Pick a cookie you like, but don't love, so you're less tempted to eat a lot of them. Instead of ice cream, indulge in low-fat frozen yogurt, (a single size portion) or a low-fat fruit smoothie. The point is to find something with just enough flavor, texture, and similarity to the food you crave to be satisfying, but healthy enough to prevent a major diet disaster.

- *Have a controlled "mini-binge" every day.* If you include a craved food in your diet, looking forward to it might help you get through the day. Just make sure that your controlled mini-binge is well planned and "safe." For example, if your mini-binge includes ice cream, plan to have a single portion in your freezer, and eat it when you are undressed and ready for bed. Your goal is to make it harder (meaning it will take work) to obtain more if your craving continues after your "mini-binge" has ended.

Neurochemicals, play a role in the development of cravings. At least 70 neurochemicals influence all aspects of behavior, including memory, appetite, cognitive functioning, mood, and sleep/wakefulness. We now know that neurochemicals affect hunger, food cravings, fullness, and satiety.

Some of the neurotransmitters and hormones that influence our eating behaviors are listed below.

Endorphins. Most people know that even moderate exercise increases endorphin production. Endorphins are responsible for the pleasure we feel when eating especially palatable foods, particularly those that are fat-filled, sweet, creamy, and highly seasoned. By giving in to our endorphin-inspired cravings, we create a vicious cycle: eating especially delicious foods increases endorphin levels further, leading us to want to eat more.

Serotonin. This is a multi-tasking neurotransmitter. High levels elevate mood, reduce anxiety, curb appetite and food cravings, increase pain tolerance, and produce restful sleep. It is synthesized in the brain from tryptophan.

Dopamine and Norepinephrine. These related neurotransmitters are produced from the amino acid tyrosine, assisted by folic acid, magnesium, and vitamin B_{12}. Both are extremely important for healthy mood, mental functioning, and alertness. Both neurotransmitters play a role in triggering desire for carbohydrates.

Neuropeptide Y (NPY) is partially responsible for intensifying cravings for carbohydrate-rich foods. Stress may increase NPY production. The stress hormone corticosterone, produced in the adrenal gland, elevates NPY production.

Neuropeptide Y is partially responsible for intensifying cravings for carbohydrate-rich foods.

Galanin. This neurochemical, along with serotonin, increases fat intake. There appears to be a direct relationship between rising galanin levels and the desire to eat foods such as ice cream, cakes, chocolate, well-marbled meats, and fried foods. Galanin production increases when body fat is used for fuel during dieting and fasting. Galanin may also stimulate carbohydrate intake.

Corticotropin-Releasing Hormone (CRH). This important hormone plays a role in reducing hunger and our desire to eat, especially during stress and dieting. When CRH is injected directly into animals' brains, they eat less; when CRH action is blocked, they eat more.

FOOD & HORMONES

Hormones—often acting in concert with neurotransmitters—are produced in other body organs and affect hunger, satiety and cravings. Some of the most important of these hormones are described below.

Insulin. Insulin, a hormone produced by pancreatic cells, is responsible for regulating blood sugar levels. Since blood sugar is probably the single most important factor controlling appetite and mood, insulin is crucial in causing food cravings.

When we eat, carbohydrates are reduced to "simple sugars," which then enter the blood stream and trigger insulin release. But carbohydrates vary in how much insulin release they trigger. Refined foods containing simple carbohydrates, such as sugary snacks or white rice, potatoes or pasta, lead to an initial release of insulin, and a drop in blood sugar levels. Eventually this decrease in blood sugar triggers hunger and more food cravings. Unprocessed foods containing complex carbohydrates (such as whole wheat bread and brown rice) break down relatively slowly, leading to gradual insulin release, and fewer cravings.

Cholecystokinin (CCK) is a hormone produced by both the brain and intestine. CCK is secreted by the intestine in response to eating. This hormone assists in digestive processes and induces feelings of satiety and sleepiness.

Cortisol is a hormone produced by the adrenal glands as part of the body's complex response to stress. Cortisol levels play a role in the proper functioning of many neurotransmitters, including serotonin, dopamine, and neuropeptide Y, consequently, it indirectly affects food cravings.

Estrogen and Progesterone are produced in the ovaries. Elevated estrogen appears to be associated with cravings for high carbohydrate/high fat foods. Estrogen levels increase during puberty and around ovulation. After ovulation, estradiol drops off and progesterone levels increase.

Testosterone is a hormone produced in the testes of men, the ovaries of women, and the adrenal glands of both. To a lesser extent than estrogen, elevated testosterone is associated with increased food intake.

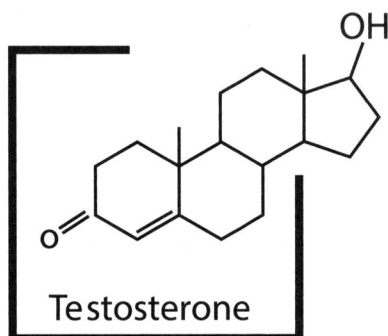

Testosterone

Leptin is a hormone produced by adipose cells. In animal studies, direct injection of leptin into the hypothalamus dramatically reduces eating. Early clinical studies on humans have found that leptin plays a complex role in eating behaviors. Leptin signals the hypothalamus to reduce food intake.

Fatty acids are produced in liver and in fat tissue. During dieting or after a long interval between meals (such as between dinner and breakfast), production of fatty acids leads to a rise in endorphins and cravings for sugar and fat-laden foods.

CHOCOLATE:
THE IRRESISTIBLE CRAVING

Most of us know that cravings for chocolate can be especially irresistible. Chocolate lovers report that when a craving for chocolate strikes, nothing else will satisfy: not lemon pie, not apple crisp, not strawberry shortcake. In fact 40% of women and 15% of men report that chocolate is the food they crave most frequently.

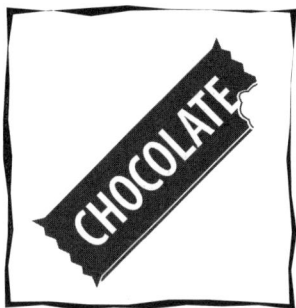

According to dietitian and author Elizabeth Somer, R.D., writing in *Food and Mood*:

Chocolate has the perfect mix of sugar and fat to turn on almost every appetite-triggering neurotransmitter. The sugar in chocolate sparks serotonin release and soothes NPY levels, contributing to the sense of well-being. The sweet taste it has also releases endorphins in the brain, giving us an immediate rush. The fat in chocolate enhances its rich flavor and aroma and satisfies galanin levels. The endorphin rush alone that is set in motion with a bite of chocolate produces a powerful pleasure sensation that is likely to be habit-forming, which might be why some people say they are addicted to chocolate.

Many chocolate foods contain both sugar and fat, but it's not just these ingredients that make chocolate so enticing. Chocolate is a complex substance containing more than 400 distinct compounds, more than twice the number in any other food. It contains theobromine and small amounts of caffeine, which provide a mental "lift" and anandamide, which is structurally similar to marijuana. According to recent research anandamide may add to chocolate's pleasure.

Chocolate is one of the few foods that is solid at room temperature and melts in the mouth, releasing aromas and flavors that both entice and satisfy. Some studies suggest that the process of seeing, smelling, and tasting chocolate plays a role in the pleasure that results from eating it.

CONTROLLING CHOCOLATE CRAVINGS

One thing is clear: if you crave chocolate, removing it entirely from your life will make you miserable. So, how can you indulge in chocolate and still lose or maintain your weight? Here are some tips:

    ∾ *Go for low-fat or low-calorie treats*. Instead of chocolate ice cream, try light ice cream, fat-free frozen yogurt, a low-calorie fudge bar, or chocolate sorbet. Experiment with different brands until you find one or two that satisfies your taste for chocolate.

~ **Drink your chocolate.** It's fairly easy to find low-fat chocolate beverages, and beverages in general reduce hunger (and sometimes cravings). Look for low-fat chocolate milk at the supermarket, or make it at home with low-fat chocolate syrup.

~ **Eat semi-sweet chocolate chips**—one at a time.

~ **Add chocolate to healthy foods and snacks.** Chocolate dipped (not drenched) strawberries, banana slices, or pineapple make a great snack.

PREGNANCY, PMS, & CRAVINGS

Food cravings during pregnancy, especially the first trimester, are legendary. Many pregnant women experience cravings for foods ranging from ice cream to pickles. Actress Julia Roberts reportedly craved French fries dipped in chocolate during her pregnancy.

Multiple factors contribute to cravings during pregnancy. Estrogen and endorphin levels are elevated, increasing cravings for carbohydrate and fat. Psychological factors probably play some role, but many questions remain and there is tremendous individual variation.

On average, women with PMS increase their caloric intake about 500 calories per day.

Premenstrual syndrome (PMS) also affects food cravings. In fact, one in three women report increased food cravings and hunger in the two weeks prior to their menstrual period. Some report consuming up to 87% more calories during this time. On average, women with PMS increase their caloric intake about 500 calories per day.

PMS symptoms are a result of hormonal changes during a woman's menstrual cycle. Research has also found that the most common symptoms of PMS, including increased cravings for sweets, coincide with reduced serotonin levels. The self-medication hypothesis may play a role in this scenario: women eat more carbohydrate-rich foods during PMS to increase serotonin levels and improve their mood. Also, endorphin levels drop off after ovulation, probably contributing to increased symptoms of depression, irritability, and anxiety, as well as elevated food cravings.

Some research suggests that refraining from craved foods may help women with PMS. When sugar and caffeine are removed from the diets of some women with PMS, their mood and energy level improve.

Can anything be done to reduce the depression, anxiety, irritability and food cravings of PMS?

There are a number of home remedies that can be helpful. Eating complex carbohydrates instead of sugary foods can cut down on food cravings. By refraining from alcohol, you can ease symptoms of depression, according to the American Academy of Family Physicians. Getting aerobic exercise and plenty of sleep—at least eight hours a night—can also boost your mood, and decrease food cravings.

If PMS and its mood swings are very severe, psychotherapy can be helpful. Discussing your feelings and concerns with a caring professional can go a long way toward reducing their intensity. Also, small doses of selective serotonin re-uptake inhibitors (SSRIs), including Prozac, Zoloft, Celexa, can help alleviate symptoms. A combination of therapy and medications may work better than either treatment alone.

EATING DISORDERS & EXTREME CRAVINGS

The high rate of food cravings among healthy people makes it clear that cravings are by no means reserved for those with eating disorders. However, extreme cravings can also play a major part in eating disorders, such as binge eating and bulimia.

Binge eating is typically defined as consuming large amounts of craved foods within a relatively short time. The definition of "large amounts of food" varies: one person may consider five cookies a binge, another, five *boxes* of cookies. Binge-eating most often takes place in secret and is accompanied by feelings of shame. Research indicates that negative mood states such as depression, anxiety, anger, and severe calorie restriction can all play a role in triggering binge-eating episodes, but hunger does not.

Quick Tips: Calming Your Cravings

Working towards moderation in eating can be daunting. However cravings do not have to defeat your weight loss efforts. Below are some tips to guide you in living healthfully with food cravings.

- *Don't give up:* Remember, your next opportunity to eat in moderation comes the very next time you put something in your mouth. Telling yourself that by giving in to a craving, you've ruined your diet for the entire day is a very common but self-defeating belief. Don't wait till tomorrow to eat with restraint again. Make your next meal a controlled one.

- *Distract yourself:* Brushing your teeth or using mouthwash when cravings strike can be a simple and surprisingly effective strategy at any time of the day or night.

- *Give in to your cravings, but not for food:* Nothing compares with the innate pleasure of eating. We are hard-wired to enjoy food and we need it to survive. To reduce food cravings and binge eating, seek out pleasurable activities instead. Make a list of enjoyable alternatives to try when a food craving strikes. Think physical pleasures: A back-rub, a foot massage, listening to music by candlelight, and getting into a Jacuzzi or sauna all provide pleasure in their own way. Sometimes even a nap makes a good substitute for an eating binge.

- *Improve your life:* The better you feel in your daily life, the easier it will be to handle food cravings. Everyone needs a strategy that reduces everyday stress. Pick a stress reducing-strategy and commit to it. A simple stroll in the park, a yoga class, playing the piano, or singing in a chorus, working in the garden, painting, crafting, needlework, and other hobbies can add to your general peace of mind and feelings of contentment.

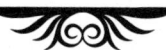

A related condition known as *bulimia nervosa* or binge-purge syndrome involves alternately eating large amounts of craved foods, and then getting rid of it before the nutrients can be absorbed. Typical purging strategies include vomiting immediately after eating and excessive laxative use. Excessive exercise, often for many hours per day at high intensity, is sometimes used to burn up calories consumed during a binge-eating episode.

THE BOTTOM LINE

Can you learn to moderate your food cravings—and, thereby, avoid gaining weight? You *can* attain weight loss by substituting healthier treats for the foods you crave, and learn to indulge in small portions of chocolate cake and premium ice cream only occasionally. To curb your cravings takes daily effort, but it's worth it.

While many of us will never attain perfection, a continued effort to moderate our intake of sugary and fatty foods will pay off with good health, increased energy, and a trim body.

Quick Tips

10 Tips to Control Cravings

1. Increase your commitment and tell friends about your goals.

2. Remind yourself of the negative long-term consequences of poor choices.

3. Enjoy the partial successes you have.

4. Distract yourself with important or pleasant tasks.

5. Don't let yourself become overextended or exhausted.

6. Replace old fattening habits with new healthy ones.

7. Keep really tempting snacks out of your house.

8. Avoid placing yourself in really tempting environments.

9. Don't let your mental and emotional resources get depleted.

10. Never go grocery shopping when you're hungry.

Chapter 7
obesity medications

"Extreme remedies are very appropriate for extreme diseases."

~ *Hippocrates, 400 B.C.*

INTRODUCTION

Everyone is looking for a "miracle pill" to counteract the obesity epidemic. But is a cure-all medicine for obesity possible? Not yet, and a magic pill is not on the horizon.

Many obesity medications, initially hyped as wonder drugs, have proven to be ineffective or to have dangerous side effects. Obesity is a complex disease that's impossible to treat with a single pill.

The Food and Drug Administration (FDA) has approved several drugs for short- and long-term treatment of obese and overweight patients with one or more other serious conditions such as heart disease, diabetes, sleep apnea, and hypertension. Most patients who receive prescriptions for obesity medications must also have tried more conventional options first: diet and exercise.

The search for a miracle pill for weight loss is big business; Americans spend over $33 billion on weight loss products/medications every year. But the track record for developing obesity medications has been poor.

Some examples of failed obesity medications are:

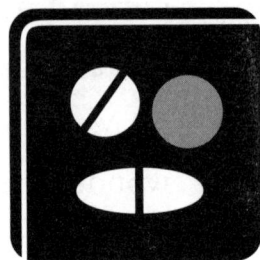

∽ Thyroid hormone, which produced weight loss by loss of lean tissues and led to cardiac arrhythmias, and sudden death.

∽ *Dinitrophenol,* which resulted in weight loss by increasing the body's metabolic rate, but caused dermatitis, liver damage, cataracts, and neuropathy.

∽ Amphetamines, which caused anorexia, addiction, and arrhythmias.

∽ Combinations of amphetamines, diuretics, thyroid hormone, and digitalis (Rainbow pills), which resulted in addiction, high blood pressure, arrhythmias, and death.

∽ Aminorex (an amphetamine analogue), which caused pulmonary hypertension.

∾ *Dexfenfluramine* combined with *phentermine* (Fen-Phen) effectively reduced weight, but was associated with valvular heart disease. The manufacturer, Wyeth-Ayerst Laboratories, voluntarily withdrew it from the market.

∾ *Phenylpropanolamine* (PPA), found in many over-the-counter appetite suppressants, was removed from the market because its use was associated with hemorrhagic stroke.

When the smoke cleared, most of the prescription medications for weight loss fell into two categories: appetite suppressants and medications that prevent the absorption of dietary fat.

FDA-APPROVED PRESCRIPTION DRUGS FOR WEIGHT LOSS

Several drugs have been approved by the FDA for weight loss *(Table 1)*. Most of these drugs are appetite suppressants and one *(orlistat)* inhibits fat absorption in the gastrointestinal tract.

Most appetite suppressants work by increasing the levels of neurotransmitters (norepinephrine

Table I

Dosages of short-term FDA-approved appetite suppressants for short-term weight loss

Agent	Dosage (mg)	Number of Times Daily
Benzphetamine	25 – 50	1 – 3
Phendimetrazine		
Short-acting	17.5 – 70	2 – 3
Long-acting	105	1
Phentermine	15 – 37.5	1
Diethylpropion		
Short-acting	25	3
Long-acting	75	1
Mazindol	1	1

Note: None of these agents are recommended for children.

and/or serotonin) in the brain by either stimulating release or inhibiting re-uptake of these substances at nerve terminals. Let's examine the properties of these anti-obesity drugs.

APPETITE SUPPRESSANTS: A SHORT-TERM SOLUTION

Appetite suppressants are only approved for short-term use (less than 12 weeks). After a few weeks of continuous use these medications lose their efficacy, making them only useful while patients learn to switch to a low-calorie diet and increase physical activity. People on appetite suppressant weight loss drugs typically lose 4 to 20 pounds when compared to placebo.

Appetite suppressants that act on norepinephrine (called noradrenergic agents) can interact with many other drugs, however, including mono-amine oxidase inhibitors (MAOI), guanethidine, central nervous system stimulants, alcohol, and tricyclic antidepressants. The effective dosages for short-term appetite suppressants are shown in *Table 1.*

Diethylpropion and *benzphetamine* are known to pass into breast milk, and all noradrenergic agents will pass into the urine and produce a positive result for amphetamine in a urine drug test.

Because these drugs increase norepinephrine levels, a neurotransmitter that constricts blood vessels and increases the heart rate, they also increase blood pressure, which must be closely monitored during treatment. If there is a sustained increase in blood pressure, the dose should be reduced or discontinued. Other possible adverse reactions are shown in *Table 2.*

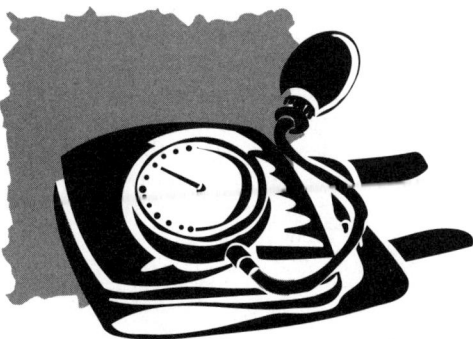

Table 2

Side effects of FDA-approved appetite suppressants for short-term weight loss

Agent	Side Effects
Benzphetamine	Blurred vision, dizziness, dry mouth, sleeplessness, stomach upset or constipation. Other side effects can include: chest pain, nervousness, pounding heart, difficulty urinating, mood changes, breathing difficulties, swelling, skin rash.
Phendimetrazine	Restlessness, anxiety, sweating, dizziness, agitation, sleeplessness, tremor, blurring of vision and rarely, psychosis. The effects on the heart include palpitations, increased heart rate and high blood pressure. Other side effects can include nausea, altered bowel habits, dryness of mouth, frequent urination and changes in libido.
Phentermine	*Phentermine* may cause dizziness, blurred vision, or restlessness, and it may hide the symptoms of extreme tiredness. It can be habit-forming. Side effects can also include increased heart rate and blood pressure, tremor, nervousness or anxiety, headache, insomnia, dry mouth, diarrhea or constipation, impotence or changes in sex drive, and rarely, hallucinations or confusion.
Diethylpropion	Restlessness or tremor, nervousness or anxiety, headache or dizziness, insomnia, dry mouth or an unpleasant taste, diarrhea or constipation, impotence or change in sex drive. *Diethypropion* can be habit-forming. Side effects can also include an irregular heartbeat or high blood pressure and rarely, hallucinations, abnormal behavior or confusion. Signs of an allergic reaction include difficulty breathing, closing of the throat, swelling of lips and tongue, and hives.
Mazindol	Dizziness, blurred vision or restlessness, nervousness, headache, dry mouth or an unpleasant taste, diarrhea, constipation, or changes in sex drive. *Mazindol* is a sympathomimetic amine, which is similar to an amphetamine. It stimulates the central nervous system, increasing the heart rate and blood pressure. Rarely, it may cause hallucinations or abnormal behavior. Taking this drug can result in psychological dependence.

WEIGHT PERFECT

Discontinuing these medications can lead to fatigue, depressed feelings, abdominal pain, nausea, vomiting, and trouble sleeping. It's also possible to regain the weight lost once the medication has been stopped. Thus, to maintain weight loss, lifestyle changes are necessary.

SIBUTRAMINE: A DRUG SURROUNDED BY CONTROVERSY

Sibutramine (Meridia), was introduced in 1997, but was taken off the market in October of 2010. Weight loss associated with this drug was modest, and the potential for increases in blood pressure and pulse was significant, as was the risk for nonfatal myocardial infarction and nonfatal stroke.

ORLISTAT: BLOCKING FAT ABSORPTION

One way to prevent weight gain is by preventing fats and other nutrients from being absorbed by the body. In the small intestine, enzymes called lipases break fats (triglycerides) down into their components (glycerol and fatty acids). The fatty acids are then collected and absorbed through the wall of the small intestine. Preventing fats from being broken down and absorbed in the intestine reduces energy input and thereby induces weight loss.

Orlistat (Xenical) is the only pancreatic and gastric lipase inhibitor approved by the FDA for long-term weight loss. *Orlistat* prevents 30% of ingested fat from being absorbed. The effective dose of *orlistat* is 120 mg three times daily or within one hour after eating fat-containing meals. While taking the drug, patients should also follow a diet that contains no more than 30% calories from fat and take a multi-vitamin supplement to prevent deficiencies in fat-soluble vitamins. A meta-analysis of clinical trials of orlistat, published in the International *Journal of Obesity and Related Metabolic Disorders*, showed that the drug produced weight loss of only 2% to 3% more than dieting alone—hardly a stellar record. *Orlistat* lowers LDL cholesterol, but its side effects can include cramping and severe diarrhea. *Orlistat* increases oxalate absorption and can increase the risk of kidney stones.

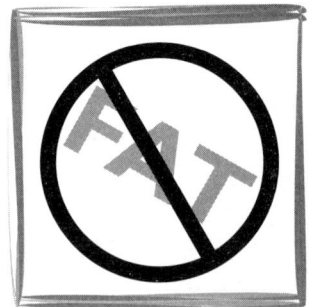

Other major side effects include gas, increased frequency and urgency of bowel movements, and oily stools. *Orlistat* is now available in a reduced dose (60 mg) and sold over-the-counter under the name Alli. Alli can still reduce absorption of fat-soluble vitamins (A, D, E, and K) and beta carotene. Patients on any form of *orlistat* should be cautious if they also take *warfarin* since decreased vitamin K absorption can increase international normalized ratio (INR) levels. The wholesale cost for a 30-day supply of Xenical/*Orlistat* is $586. A 30-day supply of Alli at wholesale is $44.

FDA-APPROVED DRUGS FOR WEIGHT MANAGEMENT

Pharmacotherapy for weight loss is reserved for adult patients with a BMI ≥30, or a BMI ≥27 and obesity-related conditions such as type 2 diabetes, hypertension, or dyslipidemia. All weight loss drugs should be avoided during pregnancy. Patients with type 2 diabetes who take drugs for weight loss may experience increased insulin sensitivity. As a result, these patients may need to reduce the dose of glucose-lowering medications to avoid hypoglycemia.

Qsymia – a combination drug containing *phentermine* and extended-release *topiramate*. This is considered the most effective weight loss drug so far (mid 2018). Qsymia produced a dose-dependent mean weight loss of 6–13 kg over 56 weeks, with little weight regression back to baseline over two years of continued use.

Side effects include dry mouth, paresthesias, constipation, dysgeusia (abnormal taste), insomnia, increased heart rate and blood pressure, and nervousness.

Problems with cognition, attention, concentration, and memory have been reported. *Phentermine* is contraindicated in patients with cardiovascular disease, hyperthyroidism, glaucoma, or a history of drug abuse.

Topirimate is an anticonvulsant and should not be stopped abruptly due to risk of seizures. It can also cause metabolic acidosis which increases the risk of kidney stones.

Qsymia is a schedule IV controlled substance. **Dosing:** 7.5/46 or 15/92 mg ER capsule. **Cost:** $186 wholesale for a 30-day supply.

Belviq or lorcaserin is a selective serotonin receptor agonist that suppresses appetite. It is a schedule IV controlled substance. Clinical trials have shown it to be only modestly effective for weight loss but it is usually well tolerated. *Lorcaserine* should be stopped if patients fail to lose ≥5% of their baseline weight by 12 weeks.

Side effects include headache, nausea, dizziness, euphoria, and problems with attention and cognition. *Lorcaserine* should not be combined with SSRIs, SNRIs, or MAOIs.

Dosing: 10 mg tablets or 20 mg ER tablets. 10 mg bid or 20 mg qd. *Cost:* $264 wholesale for a 30-day supply.

Contrave is a combination drug containing *bupropion* and *naltrexone*. *Bupropion* is a dopamine/norepinephrine reuptake inhibitor and naltrexone is a opioid receptor antagonist.

Side effects can include nausea, vomiting, headache, constipation, dizziness, and dry mouth. *Bupropion* may lower the seizure threshold and can cause CNS depression. The drug may cause increases in heart rate and blood pressure, and should not be used in patients with uncontrolled hypertension. *Naltrexone* has been reported to cause aminotransferase elevations and possible hepatotoxicity.

Dosing: 8/90 mg ER tablets given as 16/180 mg bid. *Cost:* $278 wholesale for a 30-day supply.

Saxenda or liraglutide is a glucagon-like peptide-1 (GLP-1) receptor agonist. It is given once daily by injection. *Liraglutide* is also FDA approved for type 2 diabetes as Victoza. GLP-1 receptor agnoists work by delaying gastric emptying and causing satiety.

Side effects can include nausea, diarrhea, constipation, vomiting, hypoglycemia, decreased appetite, and dyspepsia. Acute pancreatitis, gall stones, acute renal failure, and increased heart rate have been reported. Angioedema and anaphylactic reactions have occurred. *Liraglutide* is contraindicated in patients with a personal or family history of medullary thyroid cancer or Multiple Endocrine Neoplasia syndrome type 2 (MEN2).

Dosing: 18 mg/3 ml prefilled pen with usual adult dose of 3 mg SC once daily. *Cost:* $1200 wholesale for a 30-day supply.

DIET SUPPLEMENTS: THE REAL SCOOP

CHAPTER 7

From all the advertisements, you'd probably guess that diet supplements—or at least some of them—must work. Those trim, buffed "success stories" in the ads are hard to ignore. But the question of whether diet supplements are effective as weight loss aids is still controversial.

In a review study published in the *American Journal of Clinical Nutrition*, researchers Max Pittler and Edzard Ernst analyzed 30 clinical trials and review studies on 11 dietary supplements. They found little scientifically sound research supporting the effectiveness of these supplements. Some supplements also had problematic, even dangerous, side effects.

Let's look at the pros and cons of four dietary weight loss supplements: ayurvedic preparations, chromium picolinate, *Ephedra sinica*, and yerba maté.

AYURVEDIC PREPARATIONS

Ayurveda—an ancient, alternative medicine—has been practiced in India for at least 6,000 years.

In an Indian clinical study, 70 obese patients were randomly placed in four groups, including one group that received a placebo. The other groups received a variety of herbal ayurvedic preparations. The volunteers who received the ayurvedic supplements lost significant amounts of weight that ranged between 7.9 and 8.2 kg (17.4 and 18.1 pounds) compared to weight lost by the placebo group. No adverse effects were observed.

CHROMIUM PICOLINATE

Chromium is an essential trace mineral that enhances the body's use of insulin, and proponents claim it helps increase lean body mass while helping to metabolize, or "burn," carbohydrates and fats. Picolinate is a naturally occurring amino acid by-product that helps the body efficiently absorb chromium, so the two usually are paired in supplements. Chromium picolinate is supposed to help you lose weight, build lean muscle, and reduce body fat. However, there is no significant proof that the supplement affects weight loss. Claims for weight loss often are directed to obese people who may be at risk for type 2 diabetes. Again, there is no proof of weight loss or the ability to prevent diabetes. As for preventing heart disease, it's better to improve your diet, exercise, and take cholesterol-lowering drugs if appropriate.

More importantly, some in vitro and animal studies have shown that chromium induces oxidative stress, apoptotic cell death and altered gene expression, and may be carcinogenic, according to a study published in *Molecular and Cellular Biochemistry* in 2001. So the best advice is to stay with modest supplements of chromium, if you must, but the best source is food such as carrots, potatoes, broccoli, whole-grain products, and molasses.

EPHEDRA SINICA (MA HUANG)

Ephedrine is the primary active constituent of *E. Sinica*, an evergreen shrub native to central Asia. During the 1990's products containing ephedrine alkaloids (ephedra, or Ma huang) were extensively promoted as aids to lose weight, enhance sports performance, and increase energy.

Ephedra supplements have been associated with a two- to nearly fourfold risk of developing psychiatric problems, gastrointestinal symptoms, or palpitations. In April 2004, the Food and Drug Administration (FDA) prohibited the sale of dietary supplements containing ephedra. The FDA ruled that ephedra presents an unreasonable risk of illness or injury, and has been linked to significant adverse health effects, including heart attack and stroke.

YERBA MATÉ

Yerba maté has long been known as the "cowboy coffee," made by the gauchos of the immense plains, or pampas, in South America. In one clinical trial of 47 overweight patients, researchers tested a preparation of yerba maté combined with two other herbs, guarana and damiana. Both yerba maté and guarana contain large amounts of caffeine. Evidence showed that the combination preparation of yerba maté, guarana and damiana could be potentially effective in helping to decrease body weight. Guarana has some antiplatelet activity, which can be problematic in certain patients, however.

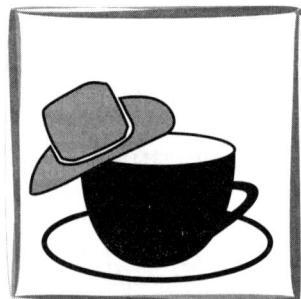

Yerba maté: the "cowboy coffee"

Other over-the-counter weight loss products can now be easily purchased at any drug store or organic food stores. These products are:

- **Diuretic compounds** – cause water loss only, not reduction of fat mass. They also result in loss of important electrolytes such as potassium, which is potentially dangerous.

- **Chitosan** – derived from the skeleton protein, chitin, found in shellfish such as shrimp and lobster. Manufacturers claim it reduces fat absorption.

- **Conjugated linoleic acid** – reported to cause weight loss, but scientific evidence shows the effects on humans are not significant.

- **Hydroxycitrate** – a substance found in the herb *Garcinia cambogia*, it may inhibit fat storage and suppress appetite. But weight loss claims have not been proven.

The pharmacologic arsenal for fighting obesity is rather meager at the moment, and many of these drugs are not as effective as clinicians or patients would like them to be. According to many researchers, the future of obesity medications will be linked to better understanding of how the body regulates weight.

HOW YOU GAIN & LOSE WEIGHT

The body has a complex system for maintaining sufficient energy and regulating weight. Neuropeptides and hormones secreted by adipose tissue and the gastrointestinal (GI) tract signal the brain's hypothalamus, telling us when and how much to eat. A few of these hormones include:

- ✺ *Leptin*—secreted by fat cells. Leptin signals the hypothalamus to suppress appetite. The more fat, the higher the leptin levels in the blood. Lower leptin levels stimulate appetite.
- ✺ *Ghrelin*—secreted by the stomach just before a meal. It provides a signal to the hypothalamus to boost appetite.
- ✺ *Peptide YY (PYY)*—secreted by the small intestine when food is present. It decreases appetite as a result of action on the hypothalamus.

These hormones may eventually provide new targets for more effective obesity drugs than ever before. However, research on new compounds that can act on appetite-regulating hormones is still in the preliminary stages.

THE BOTTOM LINE

Obesity drugs should be considered one tool that can help combat the obesity epidemic—rather than miracle pills. Because of the possibility of serious side effects, obesity drug therapy should be used only when other methods have failed, and as part of an overall weight loss effort that includes a reduced calorie diet and increased physical activity.

The history of anti-obesity medications is riddled with small successes and major failures. Many obesity drugs result in a weight loss of up to 5% when used in combination with behavioral changes. This amount of weight loss is sufficient to significantly reduce the co-morbid conditions often associated with obesity, such as hypertension, heart disease, and diabetes. But the weight loss is often temporary, and the risk of problematic side effects often outweighs the benefits.

We have a limited array of obesity medications at our disposal, and so we continue to search for more effective, longer-lasting drugs with fewer side effects. With new understanding about how our body regulates weight and energy balance, the future for treating obesity still holds some promise.

Chapter 8

devices & surgery:
the last options

"After 27 years of failure and frustration, trying every diet and exercise regimen imaginable, I weighed nearly 300 pounds. My doctor told me my health outlook was grim.

Determined to safeguard my future, I chose weight loss surgery. Sixteen months later and 155 pounds lighter, I'm healthier and happier than I've ever been."

∾ Carnie Wilson, Singer

We've all heard the stories: Carnie Wilson, who televised her gastrointestinal surgery, lost 159 pounds. Weatherman, Al Roker, had a gastric bypass procedure and lost over 100 pounds. These surgeries sound like miracles. The truth about these procedures, however, is a little more complicated.

Nine million people in the U.S. are severely obese, and thus, are candidates for weight loss surgery. Overweight is defined as a body mass index (BMI) of 25 or more, obesity, as a BMI of 30, and severe (or morbid) obesity, as a BMI of 40 or more.

Severe, or "morbid," obesity means having a body weight that is 50% to 100%, or 100 pounds, above ideal body weight.

Being morbidly obese can, and commonly does, lead to many medical problems such as:

- Arthritis
- Breast, esophageal, colorectal, endometrial, & renal cell cancer
- Cardiovascular disease
- Carpal tunnel syndrome
- Depression

- Diabetes type 2
- End stage renal disease
- Gall bladder disease
- Gout
- Hypertension
- Impaired immune and respiratory function
- Infertility
- Liver disease
- Obstetric and gynecological complications
- Pain (musculoskeletal, joint-related, heel pain)
- Sleep apnea

DEVICES FOR WEIGHT LOSS

Several devices have become available in recent years to help weight loss efforts in patients who have not succeeded with lifestyle changes. They are expensive and can be associated with significant complications and adverse effects.

Vagal Blocking device – this is a subcutaneously implanted, rechargeable neuroregulator device that blocks signals from the vagus nerve between the stomach and brain. It is intended to improve satiety and lessen food intake. Adults must have a BMI of 40–45 or a BMI of ≥ 35 and at least one comorbid obesity-related condition along with failure to lose weight during a 5-year weight loss program.

Using a laparascopic approach, the device is implanted in the thoracic side wall. Two electrodes are placed anteriorly above the gastro-esophageal junction. The electrodes are programmed to deliver high frequency electrical impulses that block normal vagus nerve signals for 9–13 hours a day.

Adverse effects include localized pain at the site of implantation, heartburn, nausea, dysphagia, belching, and abdominal pain.

Gastric Aspiration device – known as the Aspire Assist device, this procedure involves endoscopic placement of a tube into the stomach. Similar to a feeding tube with a port valve, a drainage tube and clamp, and a water reservoir, the device allows patients to drain some of their stomach contents into a toilet after eating. The overall amount of calories absorbed is reduced by approximately 30%.

Adverse effects include abdominal pain, nausea and vomiting, electrolyte imbalances, and peristomal irritation, and granulation tissue at the tube site.

Gastric Balloon devices – three gastric balloon devices have FDA approval for up to 6 months use in adults with a BMI of 30–40. Two of the devices are inserted endoscopically and filled with saline. One involves swallowing up to three deflated balloons contained in capsules. The capsule is attached to an inflation catheter which is withdrawn after the balloon is inflated. All of these devices are left in the stomach for 6 months, then deflated and removed using endoscopy. They create a sense of fullness or satiety which facilitates weight loss.

Balloon devices are contraindicated in a long list of patients: those with prior GI surgery, inflammatory bowel disease, GI ulcers, obstruction, intestinal varices, stricture or stenosis, clotting disorders, prior GI bleeds, or severe reflux.

Adverse effects include nausea, emesis, abdominal pain, reflux, distention, and bloating. A balloon can deflate, migrate, and cause GI obstruction. Complications have also included ulceration, esophageal perforation, and even death.

Gastrointestinal bypass surgery began as a treatment for cancer or severe ulcers, in which large sections of the stomach or intestine were removed. Physicians noted that patients tended to lose weight after undergoing these procedures, and began to use them to treat obesity in 1954.

The first widely used procedure in the 1960s was the intestinal bypass (jejunoileal bypass), which resulted in malabsorption. This form of bypass was eventually dropped due to unpredictable and sometimes fatal side effects, but surgeons continued to explore other types of surgery that achieved similar benefits.

Following is a look at some of the bariatric surgical procedures in use today:

BARIATRIC SURGERY: CLINICAL INDICATIONS & CONTRAINDICATIONS

Weight loss is not easy for many people. And, despite efforts to cut calories, increase exercise, and use weight loss medications, many people experience disappointing results. Any surgical procedure, however, carries a certain degree

CHAPTER 8

of risk. Clinical experience and research over the years have led to the development of guidelines for patient selection.

Indications for weight loss surgery. Before considering bariatric surgery, all potential patients should:

- ∾ Have a BMI >40 or a BMI >35 along with an obesity-related comorbidity such as diabetes, hypertension, obstructive sleep apnea, or hyperlipidemia
- ∾ Have a reasonable operative risk profile
- ∾ Have attempted all nonsurgical methods to lose weight (within reason) but without success
- ∾ Be well-informed and motivated to comply with pre-op and post-op care and instructions.

Contraindications for bariatric surgery are fairly straightforward and include:

- ∾ Current drug or alcohol abuse
- ∾ Cancer that is not in remission
- ∾ Another life-threatening illness

- An uncontrolled psychiatric disorder such as major depression, bipolar disorder, or schizophrenia
- Inability to be compliant with dietary changes, nutritional requirements such as lifelong vitamin supplementation, and follow-up care

BARIATRIC SURGERY: UNDERSTANDING THE BASICS

Surgical practice is not static. Procedures and techniques evolve over the years, based on clinical results, research, and technology. Currently, the most commonly performed procedures in the U.S. are:

- Roux-en-Y gastric bypass (RYGB)
- Sleeve gastrectomy (SG)
- Adjustable gastric banding (AGB)

Most of these procedures are done laparoscopically, which allows for a shorter recovery period and less pain than typically occurs with open surgery. Generally, these procedures have been classified as malabsorptive or restrictive based on their apparent mechanism of action causing

CHAPTER 8

weight loss. But mounting evidence demonstrates that metabolic and hormonal factors related to these procedures improve satiety and increase insulin sensitivity, thereby aiding weight loss. Changes in glucagon-like peptide-1 (GLP-1), peptide YY, and ghrelin have been documented after procedures. These neurohormonal factors seem to play an important role in the post-operative improvements in glycemic levels and resmission of diabetes.

Roux-en-Y Gastric Bypass (RYGB)

This is both a restrictive and malabsorptive procedure which creates a small (20–30 ml) proximal gastric pouch. This pouch is connected to a loop of jejunum, bypassing most of the stomach and all of the duodenum. The anastomosis site is narrow, limiting the rate of gastric emptying. The amount of food and calories that can be absorbed is greatly reduced. Bile acids and pancreatic enzymes are still able to mix with food as it passes which limits malabsorption and nutritional deficiencies. However, patients must still be followed for the possibility of deficiencies in iron, calcium, folate, vitamin B_{12}, and vitamin D. Eating foods high in sugar and fat can cause dumping syndrome (diaphoresis, dizziness, abdominal pain, nausea, and diarrhea). Some patient have developed hyperinsulinemic hypoglycemia after RYGB.

Sleeve Gastrectomy (SG)

This procedure is a laparoscopic partial gastrectomy which creates a tubular stomach passage. There are no anatomic changes to the small intestine. Since substantial and sustained weight loss occurs, SG is now performed in the U.S. as definitive treatment for severe obesity. The most serious complication involves gastric leak along the suture line which occurs in 1 to 3% of patients.

Laparascopic Adjustable Gastric Banding (AGB)

Use of this procedure has declined sharply in the U.S. in recent years. An adjustable band placed around the upper portion of the stomach restricts the volume of food a patient can eat before satiety develops. The band is usually adjusted four to six times by injecting saline via a subcutaneously placed port. Weight loss with this procedure varies and is related to the frequency of follow-up visits. Although perioperative complications and morbidity are low, over the long term, slippage, band erosion, excess vomiting, and problems with the port and tubing may require operative revision.

BILIOPANCREATIC DIVERSION WITH A DUODENAL SWITCH (BPD/DS)

This is a technically difficult procedure and now accounts for <5% of bariatric surgical procedures in the U.S. A section of the stomach is removed and the remaining section empties into the duodenum. The duodenum is resected and attached to the ileum, bypassing about 75% of the small intestine, including the sphincter of Oddi (site of entry of bile acids and pancreatic enzymes). Malabsorption and nutritional deficiencies are common.

BARIATRIC SURGERY: WHAT ARE THE BENEFITS?

Many studies have documented the physical and psychological benefits of significant weight reduction in morbidly obese patients. Depression, poor body image, and self-esteem are generally improved following weight loss surgery. In people who have gastric bypass surgery, symptoms of sleep disturbances, hypertension, cardiopulmonary problems, and gastrointestinal reflux disease often improve. Blood glucose levels typically normalize. Bariatric surgery has also been shown to have a positive impact on patients' self-image, quality of life, and overall physical activity.

SERIOUS SIDE EFFECTS & RISKS OF WEIGHT LOSS SURGERY

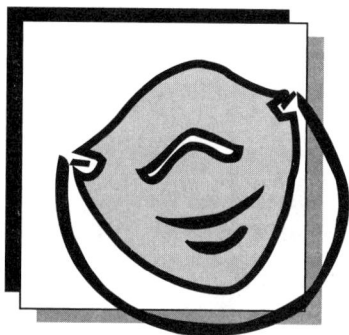

There is an approximate 10% risk of wound infection, gallstones, anastomotic leaks, stenosis, pulmonary complications, and deep venous thrombophlebitis in the short-term following bariatric surgery. In some of these cases, re-operation may be required. Overall, the most serious complications of bariatric surgery have been due to pulmonary embolism, respiratory failure, and gastrointestinal leaks, resulting in peritonitis.

Nutritional supplements must be taken to compensate for the nutrient deficiencies that occur in the first 3 to 18 months following surgery. Vomiting, and resulting protein and vitamin deficiencies, are a danger if the patient does not chew well and eat slowly. Thus follow-up by the physician is mandatory.

Depression after the first year following surgery has also been noted, according to a presentation at the annual meeting of the American College of Nutrition. Dr. George W. Cowan Jr., professor of surgery at the University of Tennessee, Memphis stated,

> *For many surgery patients, there is a belief that if they lost weight, their lives would be completely different. However, as it turns out, life's problems are not completely related to weight. So when the euphoria about the weight loss tapers off, depression sets in.*

Women of childbearing age should use effective birth control if they are undergoing weight loss surgery, as the state of malnutrition that ensues presents a possible danger to normal fetal development.

FOLLOW-UP AFTER BARIATRIC SURGERY

Long-term follow-up on a regular basis is important for every patient after bariatric surgery. Good follow-up care can ensure proper weight

Quick Tips

How to maintain weight loss after bariatric surgery

- Change your eating habits—choose foods that are nutritious and make each bite count

- Train yourself to eat more slowly

- Do not overeat—it will induce vomiting and discomfort and eventually stretch the size of the stomach pouch

- Make exercise a part of your daily routine

How to choose a bariatric surgeon

- Make sure the surgeon is a member of the *American Society of Bariatric Surgeons*

- Find out if the surgeon, and the hospital where the surgery is to be performed, is experienced in bariatric surgery

- Check to see if both the surgeon and the hospital where the surgery will be performed have appropriate resources for pre-, peri-, and post-surgical care and follow up

- Make sure there are support resources readily available to you, such as psychological and nutritional counseling and patient support groups

loss and prevent a wide array of complications. Eating habits, weight, and blood pressure are reviewed at each visit. Fasting lipid levels and HbA_{1c} are checked if they were abnormal before surgery.

Appropriate blood tests include:

ᴔ CBC

ᴔ Electrolytes

ᴔ Glucose

ᴔ BUN, Creatinine

ᴔ Albumin

ᴔ Liver function tests

Depending on the type of surgery, levels of calcium, vitamin D, B_{12}, folate, thiamine, and iron may be ordered.

Most patients should be evaluated periodically for gout, gall stones, kidney stones, hyperparathyroidism, and osteoporosis (after SG and RYGB). Diabetic patients require careful monitoring for hypoglycemia. Doses of oral hypoglycemics and insulin frequently need to be reduced and often stopped after SG or RYGB.

Finally, follow-up care should include regular screening for alcohol use and depression.

Common Psychological Effects of Weight-Loss Surgery

- self-esteem and positive emotions increase

- body image disparagement decreases

- marital satisfaction increases, but only if a measure of satisfaction existed before surgery

- healthy eating behavior is improved dramatically

IS WEIGHT LOSS SURGERY WORTH IT?

Studies have shown that the success rate for nonsurgical methods for long-term significant weight loss in morbidly obese adults is low. Most people gain all the weight lost back in the ensuing five years, and the average weight loss is only 5 pounds over a 10 to 12 week period. Failed attempts to lose weight can all result in depression, anxiety, and a preoccupation with food, all behaviors that encourage overeating and may lead to even more weight gain.

In the long run, bariatric surgery may be the most viable solution for morbidly obese people—not just because of the amount of weight that can be lost quickly, but also the health benefits that often occur after surgery. Bariatric surgery should not be undertaken lightly, as it is significant, life-changing surgery and requires life-long commitment on the part of the patient. It must also be performed by a trained surgeon who has both the resources and the time to provide all the additional care that is required for this type of surgery.

Chapter 9

the genetic puzzle: providing clues for obesity treatment

"We are not permitted to choose the frame of our destiny. But what we put into it is ours."

∾ *Dag Hammarskjöld, 1945*

INTRODUCTION

Many of us are searching desperately for ways to lose weight successfully. There are hundreds of diets, programs, gurus, and theories telling us how best to lose weight, and yet it seems to be an uphill battle. But recent research has shown that there may be a genetic connection.

Overeating is not just a failure of willpower. Obesity, in fact, is now recognized as a chronic illness. Recent research has also found that genetics and the biology of appetite play significant roles in obesity and variations in body weight.

Genetics research has already led to the development of new drugs for obesity (now in clinical trials) and may provide new targets for more effective weight loss medications.

For many people, it's hard to avoid overeating. As Jeffrey Friedman, M.D., Ph.D., of Rockefeller University said, "Food consumes our interest... To the hundreds of millions of obese and overweight individuals, it is the siren's song, a constant temptation that must be avoided lest one suffer health consequences and stigmatization."

Yet the urge to eat may not be entirely conscious. Scientists now believe it is encoded in our genes, and stimulated by the body's hormones. The system that regulates energy balance in the human body is driven to increase food intake after a significant amount of weight has been lost, for instance. Multiple hormones are the impetus behind the basic urge to eat after dieting, and combined with sensory factors, such as smell and taste, as well as emotional states, it's easy to see why many diets fail.

Researchers now believe that this primal urge to eat may be genetically determined, as well as the tendency to store calories as fat. Thus people who are

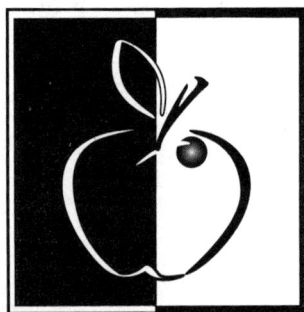

naturally lean carry genes that protect them from the consequences of overeating, whereas the obese carry genes that are throwbacks to a time of nutritional privation in which we no longer live.

James Nell proposed this idea, called the "thrifty gene hypotheses" in 1962. Thrifty genes may account for obesity in some people, as well as associated conditions, such as the metabolic syndrome. Evidence suggests that people such as the Pima Indians and Pacific Islanders, who now live a Western lifestyle but have been historically more prone to starvation, have a genotype that predisposes them to store energy as fat. Once they leave behind their traditional rural lifestyle— one of nutritional privation—and are exposed to a traditional Western diet and sedentary lifestyle, they have a high risk for obesity and its complications. Thus, they're more likely to develop glucose intolerance and diabetes as well as the metabolic syndrome.

A study of 432 Japanese-Americans from 68 families published in *Diabetes* provided more proof that the metabolic syndrome and its risk factors—including obesity—are highly heritable.

The researchers found that body fat; blood lipids, insulin and glucose levels; blood pressure and C-reactive protein values (higher values signal inflammation and an increased risk of heart disease) were significantly influenced by genetics.

At least 40% of variation in body fat is thought to be attributable to genetic factors. Genes are also responsible for more than 60% of the variation in abdominal obesity in postmenopausal women.

GENES & BMI: HOW STRONG A CONNECTION?

Studies of twins provided the first proof of a link between obesity and genes in humans. In 1990, psychiatrist Albert Stunkard, M.D., and his colleagues at the University of Pennsylvania in Philadelphia studied 311 pairs of twins who were reared apart (93 identical and 213 fraternal) and 362 pairs of twins who were reared together (154 identical and 208 fraternal) in a study published in the *New England Journal of Medicine.* They found high correlation between the BMIs of identical twins whether

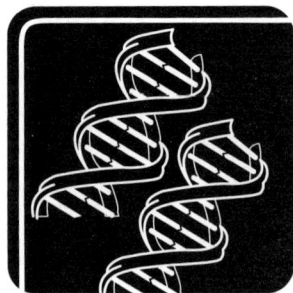

they were reared together or apart. Stunkard's group concluded that genetic factors were more important than environmental factors in developing obesity.

Other research by Hermine Maes, Ph.D., revealed that genetic factors explained 67% of the variability in BMI among family members. In her 1997 study, published in the journal *Behavioral Genetics*, Dr. Maes compared more than 25,000 pairs of twins and 50,000 family members, both biological and adoptive, and noted BMI for different family groups. She found that identical twins had the most similar body weights, followed by fraternal and non-twin siblings. There was little similarity between spouses or adoptive family members.

The findings of Maes' group, as well as Stunkard's group, clearly point to hereditary or genetic influences on obesity.

OF MICE & MEN: NEW GENETIC DISCOVERIES

Studies on mice through the years have also given us important insights into how genes can help cause obesity.

From 1902 through the 1990s, several strains of genetically obese mice have been documented. In the 1950s, a mutant mouse strain called the *ob* mouse was bred at Jackson Laboratories in Bar Harbor, Maine. When a mouse inherits two copies of the *ob* gene, it weighs as much as five times its normal counterpart.

The *ob* mouse has a metabolic defect in the ability to generate heat, a condition that is instrumental in helping cause obesity. By the time it is weaned at 21 days, the ob mouse becomes obese and hyperphagic (it eats three times more food than a normal mouse).

THE BIOLOGY OF APPETITE

Research over the past 20 years also shows strong evidence that there are genetic influences on the complex system of hormones that control our appetites.

One of the most important advances in understanding the genetics of obesity came in 1994, when a research team at Rockefeller University, New York, discovered a hormone called leptin.

Leptin is the primary hormone that regulates long-term storage of body fat (or body weight). Leptin is produced by adipose cells, and signals the hypothalamus how much fat is stored in the body. Leptin signals the hypothalamus to shut off appetite when body fat stores are high.

The researchers at Rockefeller University found that mice that had been genetically engineered not to produce leptin became morbidly obese, and these same mice lost weight if they were given leptin supplements.

In humans, researchers have found similar cases of genetic leptin deficiency.

A 1997 study of two severely obese Pakistani children, who were cousins, turned up the first cases of leptin deficiency in humans. Stephen O'Rahilly, M.D., an expert in metabolic abnormalities, found that the children—who were hyperphagic as well as morbidly obese—had no leptin in their blood at all. At age eight. the girl weighed 190 pounds and the 2-year-old boy, 165 pounds. Further testing of DNA from their fat tissue, and the DNA of 10 family members, turned up a mutation that was homozygous (both genes were defective) in the children and heterozygous (one gene was normal, one was defective) in their four parents. Dr. O'Rahilly's research has been published in a series of papers since 1997.

Dr. O'Rahilly treated the children with leptin, and the effect was instantaneous. They were able to eat normal meals and no longer constantly thought

leptin therapy can have a significant effect on hyperphagia in some patients.

about food. Their weight slowly decreased over the following year. Later research has shown that leptin therapy can have a significant effect on hyperphagia in some, but not all, patients.

Since the late 1990s, scientists have uncovered other cases of obesity caused by either congenital leptin deficiency or a mutation in the gene that encodes the body's receptor for leptin. A receptor is a protein that must bind to a hormone (such as leptin) before a cellular response can occur.

Despite the success of leptin replacement therapy, it is far from the answer to obesity. Obesity caused by leptin deficiency appears to be extremely rare in human populations; in fact there have only been 12 documented cases. Dr. Friedman says, "It appears that the intrinsic sensitivity to leptin is variable and that, in general, obese individuals are leptin-resistant. Because of this, only a subset of obese people respond to leptin therapy with a significant amount of weight loss; the majority do not."

Though leptin deficiency is rare, the response of some patients to leptin therapy has provided important proof of the biological function of leptin in controlling appetite in humans.

Research also indicates that leptin affects the gene expression and pathways of other appetite suppressing and appetite-stimulating hormones— which may soon be targets for new drug therapies for obesity. These include the hormones PYY and ghrelin, proteins that help regulate food intake and body weight. Research indicates there may be promising treatments that target PYY and ghrelin—treatments that may help curb appetite and aid weight loss.

CAN SINGLE GENE DEFECTS CAUSE OBESITY?

Are there other single gene defects that can cause obesity? The answer appears to be yes. In addition to leptin deficiency, the following single gene mutations have also been linked to obesity, but findings in human subjects are limited at present:

∾ POMC deficiency

∾ MC4R deficiency

In 2010, a gene that increases the risk of obesity and Alzheimer's disease was identified. Called FTO (fat mass and obesity gene), it also increases the risk of atrophy in the frontal and occipital lobes of the brain. Research suggests the effects of the gene can be minimized by a low-fat diet and regular exercise.

PRO-OPIOMELANOCORTIN (POMC) DEFICIENCY

Dr. Heike Krude and her colleagues at Humboldt University in Berlin have found that children with a mutation affecting pro-opiomelanocortin (POMC) suffer from severe obesity. Her findings were published in 1998 in *Nature Genetics*. Adults with a POMC genetic mutation typically show elevated levels of POMC, a hormone that affects the secretion of cortisol and epinephrine from the adrenal gland, as well as food intake. Patients can exhibit severe childhood obesity, abnormal glucose homeostasis, elevated levels of proinsulin, hypogonadotropic hypogonadism and hypocortisolemia. Though research on POMC mutations is in the initial stages, studies do show that POMC is important for energy homeostasis—knowledge that could eventually lead to treatments for this phenotype.

MC4R DEFICIENCY

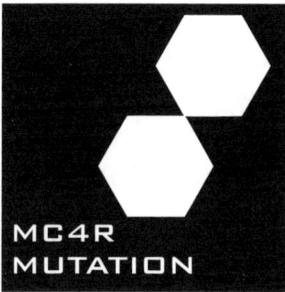

MC4R
MUTATION

Melanocortin 4 receptor (MC4R) is a gene related to appetite suppression, and several research groups have found mutations in this gene. People with the MC4R mutation can be severely obese and most exhibit hyperphagia and binge eating.

As well as increased fat mass, subjects with MC4R can also display an increase in lean mass. MC4R deficient patients usually have severe hyperinsulinemia, and increased bone mineral density and linear growth.

The severity of symptoms of those with MC4R mutations, however, tends to ameliorate over time. Obese adult patients with the mutation show less intense hunger and are less hyperinsulinemic than children with the same mutation.

The most significant aspect of the MC4R mutation is its effect on eating behavior. In a study published by Branson et al in the *New England Journal of Medicine* in 2003, researchers found that out of 469 severely obese adult subjects, 24 had MC4R mutations. All the carriers were binge eaters as opposed to 14% of obese subjects who did not have an MC4R mutation.

Another study published by Farooqi et al, also in the *New England Journal of Medicine* in 2003 found of 500 children with severe childhood obesity, 6% had MC4R mutations. The energy consumed at an ad libitum meal by carriers of the MC4R mutation was three times that of siblings who were not carriers. The researchers also found that in some *binge-eating disorder is usually predictive of poor outcomes in the treatment of obesity.*

families with an MC4R mutation, environmental influences had some impact on the development of obesity.

The researchers concluded that MC4R does have a critical role in controlling eating behavior and fat mass in human beings.

Since binge-eating disorder is usually predictive of poor outcomes in the treatment of obesity, such as gastric surgery, MC4R mutations could be one cause of treatment failure. However, more research is needed on this question.

OBESITY GENES: HERE, THERE & EVERYWHERE

It is important to remember that most genetic obesity disorders occur in only a small percent of the population. The vast majority of obesity cases are due to the interactions of multiple genes (polygenic inheritance), as well as lifestyle and environmental influences. We now know that there are more than 100 genes or specific sites on genes that could potentially influence obesity. Research is focusing on which genes or genomic regions modulate the human response to diet.

There are no special diets for people with monogenic disorders for obesity. However, as we learn more about how genes interact with diet, doctors may be able to prescribe individualized nutrition plans to prevent or manage chronic disease conditions, including obesity. This is the basis of a new field of study called *nutritional genomics*. Although it is not yet ready for medical practice, this science holds promise for eventually using nutritional therapies to treat obesity and other disorders.

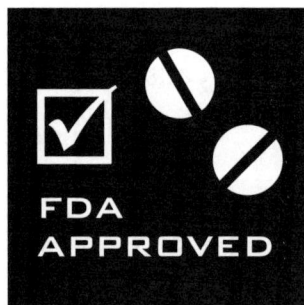

FDA APPROVED

THE BOTTOM LINE

Obesity is not a simple disease, but rather a complex condition with genetic and nutritional components. Researchers have used genetics in animal and human models to get a better, but still incomplete, picture of the molecular basis of the disease.

According to Jeffrey Friedman, M.D., Ph.D., writing in the journal *Science*:

Our approach to the obesity epidemic should be analogous [to cancer research]; identify the molecular components of the system that regulates body weight, define what is different about the system in lean and obese subjects, and elucidate how environmental and developmental factors alter the function of this system. Such a foundation is essential for the development of rational therapies.

To this end, the new tools of genomic sciences will help scientists identify the genes associated with obesity, establish the importance and interactions of those genes, and design new diagnostic tests, drug treatments and nutritional therapies for genetic obesity.

CHAPTER 9

Chapter 10
fit for life

"If we could give every individual the right amount of nourishment and exercise, not too little and not too much, we would have found the safest way to health."

    ∾ *Hippocrates, Greek physician (c.460–c.370 B.C.)*

"Those who think they have not time for bodily exercise will sooner or later have to find time for illness."

    ∾ *Edward Stanley, 19th Century English poet and politician*

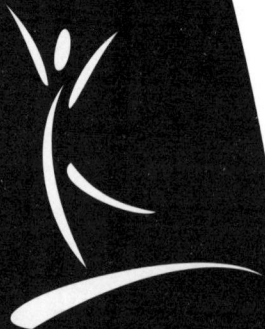

The value of regular exercise has been extolled since ancient times, and the number of known benefits continues to increase with each new study on the topic. Being physically active can:

- Reduce the risk of heart disease, stroke, and diabetes
- Reduce blood pressure
- Keep bones, muscles, and joints healthy
- Reduce anxiety and depression
- Protect against falling, osteoporosis, and bone fractures in the elderly
- Reduce pain and joint swelling from arthritis
- Improve sleep
- Lower cholesterol levels
- Protect against breast and colon cancer
- Reduce the risk of colds
- Reduce the severity of menstrual cramps and hot flashes
- Reduce the risk of Alzheimer's and vascular dementia

One of the most important aspects of physical activity is its positive effect on weight loss and maintenance. Losing weight plays a large part in decreasing the risks of chronic diseases, and improving the function of vital organs.

In this chapter we'll talk about how exercise benefits those in different age groups, the pros and cons of different types of exercise, and how to most easily maintain an exercise habit.

ARE WE ALL COUCH POTATOES?

Despite our wealth of knowledge about diet and exercise, and the American obsession with losing weight, 60% of adults do not get enough exercise. Twenty five percent do not get any exercise at all, according to the Centers for Disease Control (CDC). And one half of children in grades 9 to 12 do not get regular, vigorous, exercise.

A great deal of emphasis is placed on the type of foods to eat to achieve weight loss—low-fat, low-carbohydrate, vegetarian—but the role of exercise in weight loss, and maintaining weight, is just as important.

As well as helping burn calories, including exercise in a weight-loss program ensures that the body draws from stored fat, rather than muscle, for

Calorie Burn for 30 Minutes

Activity	150 lbs.	200 lbs.	250 lbs.
Walking (2 mph)	102	138	174
Walking (4 mph)	186	246	306
Running (5 mph)	322	429	534
Running (7 mph)	423	561	696
Badminton	162	225	282
Basketball	210	282	351
Cycling (5 mph)	150	201	249
Cycling (13 mph)	318	426	534
Dancing	125	165	207
Racquetball	270	351	432
Skiing (downhill)	288	384	480
Skiing (x-country)	354	471	582
Squash	270	351	432
Swimming	115	153	192
Tennis	204	276	345
Volleyball	162	225	486

the energy it needs. In addition, exercise builds muscle tissue, which burns calories faster than body fat, and also strengthens muscles and reduces inches. Psychologically, exercise is important for relieving stress and tension, and also promotes a feeling of self-confidence, which can lead to improved self-image and mood.

CHAPTER 10

CHILDREN & ADOLESCENTS: TOO MUCH SCREEN TIME, NOT ENOUGH EXERCISE

The CDC reports that almost half of American children aged 12 to 21 years do not engage in regular vigorous exercise, and 14% of young people reported no recent physical activity. Too much time spent in front of the computer, TV, and video games, in addition to unhealthy diets, have caused the number of overweight children to increase astronomically.

Almost 13% of 6- to 11-year-olds are obese. Overweight and obesity in adolescents is rising rapidly, and is becoming a significant health problem. Adolescents are becoming increasingly sedentary, which is a key contributing factor to the rising rates of obesity in this group. Studies have shown that less than 60 minutes per day of vigorous physical activity in children aged 11 to 15 can lead to overweight.

The health implications of obesity in the young can be enormous. The American Diabetes Association notes an increase in the occurrence of type 2 diabetes among American children, particularly in African American, Latino, and

Native American children. In children regular exercise decreases the risk of diabetes, heart disease, high blood pressure, and other chronic disorders. The fact that it helps control weight can also have a significant effect on a child's self-esteem and confidence, and can encourage healthy socialization. Exercise also leads to better sleep.

Acquiring good exercise habits in childhood will benefit a child later in life. Children who get 35 to 60 minutes of walking or other exercise every day will have stronger bones, lungs, and hearts, and are much more likely to continue their exercise habits into adulthood, with life-enhancing and life-prolonging effects.

WHY IS EXERCISE VITAL IN MIDDLE AGE?

The more we age, the more we're prone to developing chronic conditions and disorders. Following a healthy lifestyle that includes good nutrition and exercise can go a long way in preventing disease and disability. During middle age, the adult metabolism naturally begins to slow

CHAPTER 10

down, and it can become more difficult to keep off extra weight.

Remaining physically active can be key in keeping off those extra pounds, and reducing risk for the chronic diseases associated with being overweight.

MENOPAUSE: HOW EXERCISE HELPS

One of the unfortunate effects of menopause is a tendency toward weight gain and increased waist circumference (the dreaded apple shape), both known to be risk factors for cardiovascular disease. But this tendency can be countered. Data from the Women's Healthy Lifestyle Project showed that initiating lifestyle changes including a healthy diet and regular exercise in the premenopausal years significantly reduces or prevents both weight gain and increased waist circumference.

Another health problem that crops up in middle age and worsens with increasing age is osteoporosis. This condition causes a decrease in bone mass (up to 20% in the five to seven years following menopause), resulting in fragile bones and a predisposition to hip and spine fractures.

Osteoporosis

Facts & Figures

- In the United States, more than 40 million people either already have osteoporosis or are at high risk due to low bone mass.

- Age increases the risk of osteoprosis. Bone loss builds up over time, and bones become weaker with advancing age.

- About one in five hip fracture patients over age 50 die in the year following their fracture as a result of associated medical complications.

Source: National Institute of Arthritis and Musculoskeletal and Skin Diseases (NIAMS). Osteoporosis: Handout on Health. Available at: *http://www.niams.nih.gov/Health_Info/Bone/Osteoporosis/osteoporosis_hoh.asp.* Accessed August 9, 2018.

Exercise is vital in preventing osteoporosis. The Bone, Estrogen and Strength (BEST) study, found that postmenopausal women who performed regular aerobic, resistance, and weight-bearing exercise experienced an improvement in bone mineral density (BMD), whether or not they were taking hormone replacement therapy.

CHAPTER 10

Regular exercise decreases mortality and morbidity in older adults and results in improved cardiovascular, endocrine, metabolic, and psychological health even when exercise is not initiated until age 75. Exercise helps preserve bone density in post-menopausal women, improves balance, and thus decreases the risk of falls and fractures. Exercise can help reduce pain and improve function in osteoarthritis, and reduces the incidence and severity of type 2 diabetes.

The National Institute of Arthritis and Musculoskeletal and Skin Diseases (NIAMS) advises a gradual exercise program, particularly one involving strengthening and range of-motion exercises, to help improve or maintain joint function and pain. Strengthening exercises help increase support for the joints by building up surrounding muscle. Exercises aimed at tightening

Strengthening exercises help increase support for the joints by building up surrounding muscle.

the muscles can be undertaken even by individuals who have inflammation and pain. Joint stiffness can be eased and flexibility and movement improved by range of motion exercises. In the case of back pain, exercises that stretch and extend the back can be significant in preventing long-term disability.

As well as aerobic exercise, strength training is important for older adults. Sarcopenia (the loss of muscle mass) can result in a 15% to 30% loss of strength per decade in adults age 50 and older. For the elderly, an increase in strength means an increase in independence. The ability to walk, lift and climb stairs are often significantly improved with exercise. This improvement can lead to a better quality of life, which in turn helps reduce the occurrence of depression and feelings of uselessness in older adults.

Both yoga and T'ai Chi Chuan are good forms of exercise for older adults. Both involve slow movement, are easy on the joints, and can be performed at several levels of intensity. Aquatic exercise is also recommended for the elderly, as it is gentle on the weight-bearing joints. Walking,

CHAPTER 10

swimming, and balance and flexibility exercises are also beneficial.

Senior centers often offer exercise programs, and many have trained geriatric exercise counselors or personal trainers who can provide advice about appropriate forms of exercise. Physical therapists are also helpful in identifying areas of concern and designing a program that takes physical limitations into account. Most older people can participate in aerobic and resistance programs if they undertake a program that gradually increases in intensity. Previously sedentary individuals should begin with 5- to 10-minute periods of moderate physical activity, such as walking, and gradually increase the amount of time spent exercising. Muscle-strengthening exercises are also very beneficial as they help prevent falls and improve the ability to perform the tasks of daily life.

Before beginning an exercise program, older patients should consult with their physicians. It is the responsibility of physicians to encourage physical activity on a regular and ongoing basis. Data shows that a physician's advice is strongly taken to heart by older patients.

People with disabilities may believe physical activity is not appropriate for them. Yet exercise can provide some of them with many health benefits. Many may still be capable of improved muscle strength and stamina, reduction in high blood pressure, or decrease in the incidence of heart disease or diabetes associated with activity.

Studies have shown that exercise does not need to be strenuous to achieve health benefits. For

exercise does not need to be strenuous to achieve health benefits.

instance, 30 to 40 minutes of wheeling oneself in a wheelchair can often provide moderately intense exercise. The type of activity performed can often be adjusted to accommodate the individual's particular disability, and still provide significant health benefits.

People with disabilities should get their physician's advice on how to start an exercise program, good types of exercise, and what the objectives of their exercise program should be.

CHAPTER 10

Physical and occupational therapists can be immensely helpful here.

HOW MUCH EXERCISE IS ENOUGH?

Moderate-intensity physical activity is important for a healthy lifestyle, and is achievable for people of nearly all ages and levels of fitness. Exercise—even exercise aimed at achieving weight loss does not have to be grueling to produce results. Most people, regardless of age can benefit from a more active lifestyle.

Exercise greatly enhances weight loss efforts. Many clinicians recommend moderate aerobic exercise every day for periods of 30 minutes or more for good health and weight loss. Yet some studies show long-term weight loss requires 60 minutes of exercise five times a week.

In a randomized controlled study called STRRIDE, published in the *Archives of Internal Medicine*, researchers studied the effects of exercise on previously sedentary, overweight men and women aged 40 to 65 years. They found that even a small amount of moderately intense exercise (such as walking 30 minutes each day) in subjects who made no attempt to diet produced both weight loss and a reduction in body fat.

Moderate-intensity physical activity is an activity that burns 3.5 to 7 calories per minute (kcal/min); examples would be walking briskly, mowing the lawn, dancing, swimming, or bicycling. Vigorous-intensity physical activity is any activity that burns 7 calories per minute; examples would be jogging, swimming laps, high-impact aerobics, or bicycling uphill.

CHOOSING THE RIGHT EXERCISE PROGRAM

A comprehensive physical activity routine includes three kinds of activities:

- ∾ Aerobic Exercise
- ∾ Strength Training
- ∾ Flexibility Exercises

AEROBIC EXERCISE: (BICYCLING, WALKING, SWIMMING, AEROBIC DANCING)

Aerobic exercise increases heart rate, works muscles, and raises respiratory rate. A total of 30 minutes a day, five days a week, is a good regimen for most people to stay in shape. For the couch potatoes among us, walking five to 10 minutes a day is a great way to start, and this can be gradually increased as one's fitness level improves. When trying to lose weight, walking longer than 30 minutes or adding additional exercise to the routine is beneficial.

BICYCLING

People used to walk and cycle everywhere, but the car is the transportation method of choice for Americans for even short distances. Yet, bicycling can have enormous cardiovascular benefits, as well as resulting in significant weight loss. Instead of driving to the store or a friend's house, try biking. If you have access to a park, bike there on the weekends. And in cold, rainy weather, a stationary bike can provide the same benefits. There are many bicycle clubs, and joining one can have social as well as physical benefits.

WALKING

Walking is one of the best overall types of exercise. It is easy to do, can be performed at any pace, requires only a good pair of walking shoes, and has great aerobic benefits. To start, you should walk slowly for five minutes, and then speed up the pace over the next five minutes. Follow this with a cooldown walk of an additional five minutes. Stand up straight, swing your arms, and maintain a steady pace. Do at least three 15-minute walks per week to start, and gradually increase the brisk walking portion by two to three minutes per week. As you become accustomed to walking regularly, pick up the pace and walk farther. Walking with a friend can make the walk more enjoyable and encourage you to stick to a regular schedule.

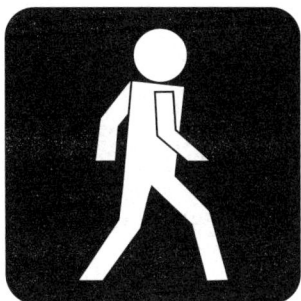

WEIGHT TRAINING • STRENGTHENING • RESISTANCE TRAINING
(Lifting weights, using resistance bands, doing push ups or sit ups)

Strength or weight training increases strength, builds and tones muscles, increases endurance, and is particularly beneficial to people over 50 years of age. It can be an important contributor to weight loss since it helps maintain lean body mass.

CHAPTER 10

It increases bone density, which decreases the risk of osteoporosis, improves coordination and balance, and can help prevent muscle injury. Once you have learned how a particular exercise is done, you should choose a weight that allows you to do the exercise 8 to 12 times for one to two sets.

Weight training should be undertaken two to three times a week, with a day's rest between sessions to allow muscles to recover. It should be performed in addition to aerobic exercise such as walking, swimming, or aerobic classes to most effectively burn calories and decrease the risk of cardiovascular disease.

FLEXIBILITY EXERCISES: STRETCHING

Stretching is important as a warm-up prior to exercise to help prevent injury. When joints are flexible, they can also move through a greater range of motion with less energy. Stretching decreases resistance in the tissues, thus protecting against overextending muscles and other tissues during exercise. Slow, static stretching (gradual elongation of the muscle that is held in the furthest comfortable position without pain for 15 to

30 seconds) can help reduce muscle soreness after exercise. Stretching can reduce the amount of effort needed to achieve and maintain good posture in the activities of daily living by helping to realign soft tissue structures.

SWIMMING

Swimming involves almost all the muscles in the body, and exercises them with less stress than working out on land. Yet the resistance provided by moving through water increases the amount of work the muscles have to perform, and helps to strengthen them. Also, swimming can provide some protection for arthritic or damaged joints, and it is also excellent cardiovascular exercise.

AQUATIC EXERCISE

Like swimming, aquatic exercise can be extremely beneficial, particularly for the elderly, people with disabilities, people with injuries, and for those who have not worked out for a long time. The water provides buoyancy for the limbs, while also providing extra resistance, and thus can help build muscle and joint strength. According to the Arthritis Foundation, water aerobics are as beneficial as land aerobics for health, but protect the joints. Studies show that a healthy person can burn 400 to 700 calories per hour in the water, depending on size, exercise intensity, and cardiovascular condition. Water exercise provides a fitness avenue even for individuals with severely restricted range of motion or who experience too much pain for land-based exercise.

YOGA

There are many forms of yoga, and some are quite strenuous. Hatha, one of the most popular types of yoga, is a gentle form of exercise that can decrease blood pressure, pulse rate, and respiratory rate, while improving cardiovascular and respiratory efficiency. It also increases musculoskeletal flexibility and range of motion of the joints. It can have a positive effect on posture, balance, strength, and endurance. Doing yoga tends to improve sleep and boost the immune system. It is a particularly good form of activity for the elderly and people who are not able to do strenuous exercise. Surprisingly enough, yoga also tends to normalize weight. In addition, the psychological effects are numerous. Improved mood, increased self-actualization, decreased hostility, and a sense of well-being are common benefits. A single yoga class has actually been demonstrated to reduce cortisol levels!

T'AI CHI

Like yoga, T'ai chi involves the performance of slow, deliberate movements that gently tone muscles and increase flexibility. Some evidence suggests this ancient Chinese form of exercise also boosts immune system capacity. It stimulates the central nervous system, lowers blood pressure, and enhances blood circulation. Patients with congestive heart failure (CHF) who practiced T'ai chi twice a week had substantial improvements in quality of life, overall mood, and cardiac exercise self-efficacy. T'ai chi also helps reduce stress, increases energy, and improves balance and coordination. Most experts agree that T'ai chi can offer important health benefits, particularly for

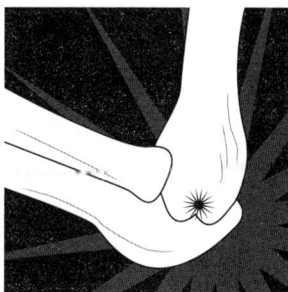

CHAPTER 10

older adults. Studies show that practicing T'ai chi regularly may slow cardiorespiratory decline and provide suitable aerobic exercise for the elderly. It has been shown to reduce the number of falls in patients with Parkinson's disease.

HOME EXERCISE: MAKE IT INVITING

Working out at home may be a more convenient way to exercise, but it requires as much commitment as going to the gym. It is easy to become distracted, make excuses, or postpone exercising when you are in the comfort of your home. But if going to the gym is difficult due to scheduling conflicts, lack of transportation, or other reasons (like being a recluse who doesn't like comparing herself to 20-somethings with perfect bodies), working out at home may be a good solution.

It's best to set aside a room for exercising, if possible, and the space must be large enough to accommodate whatever equipment you'll use. Making the environment inviting will help encourage regular use of exercise equipment, and ready access to a television or stereo will help counteract boredom. The room should have

Tips for Keeping Motivated to Exercise

- Find an exercise buddy and encourage and support each other

- Make a specific exercise plan and stick to it (ie, walk on Monday, aerobics on Tuesday, swimming on Wednesday, etc)

- Keep a log of your progress, including weight loss and body fat measurements

- Change your fitness program as your strength and endurance increase to provide a challenge

- Reward yourself periodically for sticking with it

How to Be Active When You Have a Busy Lifestyle

- Climb the stairs instead of taking the elevator

- Park a little farther away from your office or home and walk

- Get off the bus or subway a stop or two early and walk.

- Take a walk after dinner instead of watching TV

- Play with your kids or pets

- Dance to the radio while doing chores

carpeting, or there should be mats spread on the floor to cushion impact.

EXERCISE EQUIPMENT

What equipment should you choose for an exercise room? It's really a matter of preference and budget. Anything from a jump rope and dumbbells, exercise DVDs, or a variety of machines, including a treadmill, rowing machine, Pilates, etc., will do the trick. The American College of Sports Medicine provides recommendations on line for various types of exercise equipment. The equipment must be effective, well-constructed, and above all, safe.

DON'T BE A COUCH POTATO: GET UP & MOVE!

Making exercise a habit can be challenging, but it can be accomplished. Choose a form of exercise that you love doing, because you will be more likely to make a habit of it. Dancing, swimming, bicycling, and playing sports are all forms of exercise that can be enjoyable pursuits in themselves—and can actually make exercise fun.

Couch Potatoes

Tips on starting and maintaining regular exercise if you have not been active for a long time:

- Start with more gentle exercise such as walking.

- Slowly increase the pace and the length of time you exercise as you become stronger.

- Remember, even a few minutes of exercise a day will make a difference until you reach the recommended goal of 30 minutes a day.

- Pick an activity you enjoy, such as swimming or dancing.

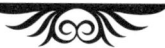

Set aside a certain time period every day for exercise, and don't let anything keep you from it. Remember this is something you are doing for yourself. Exercise classes are a good idea, as they provide a consistent schedule, and some expert guidance.

If you choose to walk, do so inside a mall during the colder months or when the weather is inclement. Exercise DVDs and online programs are also useful if you prefer to exercise at home. Many video programs include exercisers of all body sizes—which can be a boost for your

How to Avoid Exercise-Induced Injury

- Start slowly and increase your pace gradually.

- Monitor your heart rate and level of fatigue.

- Be aware of any physical discomfort.

- Be aware of breathlessness and muscle soreness— these could be signs of overexertion.

- Be aware of signs of a heart attack, including sweating, arm and chest pain, dizziness, light-headedness, and nausea.

- Use the appropriate equipment and wear appropriate clothing. ·

- Warm up your muscles for three to five minutes prior to exercising. ·

- Cool down by decreasing your level of activity over a 3 to 5 minute period.

- Drink a glass of water before beginning, and drink a half cup of water every 15 minutes you are exercising.

- Don't exercise outside in extremes of weather or air pollution.

- Put the devices away and focus on the activity at hand.

Source: The National Center for Chronic Disease Prevention and Health Promotion. Nutrition and Physical Activity. What are some tips for avoiding activity-induced injuries?

self-esteem—and they're fairly easy to follow, even if you have two left feet or have been previously sedentary. Recruiting a buddy to exercise with you regularly will also help you stay with your exercise routine, and bolster your social life as well.

When making an exercise plan, set realistic short-term and long-term goals, and stick to them. Keep an exercise log and note your progress, and reward yourself for your successes. Start slowly and gradually increase the amount of time you spend exercising as your strength and endurance increase. Above all, keep in mind the psychological benefits of exercise. The endorphins generated by exercise may actually make it a habit you won't want to give up.

THE BOTTOM LINE: EXERCISE MATTERS

There is a health crisis in the United States that can be individually addressed by improving our fitness levels. Two thirds of Americans are overweight, and one third are obese, partly due to diet, but also because of our sedentary lifestyle.

Regular physical activity reduces the risk of heart disease, depression, diabetes, Alzheimer's,

How to Burn Off a Big Mac

Nutritionists in Britain calculated how far you'd have to walk to burn off a typical Big Mac meal—a Big Mac, fries, and a milkshake, totaling 1411 calories. Their answer? You'd need to walk 9.5 miles to shake off all that fat and calories. To ward off the extra fat and calories in a meat pizza meal (930 calories), you'd have to walk for 6.2 miles. However, burning off the 45 calories in an apple is easy—and only requires a stroll of .3 miles.

colon cancer, high blood pressure, and possibly stroke. It builds healthy joints, bones and muscles; helps relieve arthritis pain and inflammation; can reduce anxiety and depression and improve self-esteem. Exercise also controls weight and thus can be instrumental in preventing or improving the symptoms of many chronic diseases that are associated with obesity. The Cardiovascular Health Study which enrolled nearly 6,000 Americans ages 65 and older found that a sedentary lifestyle alone accounted for about 25% of the risk of heart-related deaths in depressed people.

Moderate, regular exercise of only 30 minutes daily is enough to provide weight loss and health benefits. And it's never too late, or too early, to begin a physically active lifestyle. Children who are taught the value of exercise will be less likely to become overweight and will develop strong, healthy bodies. They'll also be less prone to chronic illnesses such as heart disease and diabetes. Research has shown that beginning exercise even over the age of 75 has significant health benefits.

We don't need to stay stuck in a sedentary lifestyle. Once we get moving, we can improve our health, lose weight, and generally enhance our quality of life.

Chapter 11

weight perfect:
optimal weight for life

"I've been on a diet for two weeks and all I've lost is 14 days."

～ *Totie Fields*

"The one way to get thin is to reestablish a purpose in life."

～ *the late Cyril Connolly, writer, editor, and book reviewer*

Most dieters know that maintaining weight loss can be difficult. In fact, you've probably heard that it's well nigh impossible. But scientific evidence now reveals that maintaining weight loss for years—or even a lifetime—is achievable. In fact, thousands of people have done it successfully.

Most people who maintain long-term weight loss have discovered effective strategies that keep them motivated and dedicated to healthy lifestyle habits. This chapter will show you the many resources and behavioral tools that can help you achieve long-lasting weight loss.

In the end, the payback is worth it—in terms of improved health, more self-confidence, and a happier outlook on life.

HOW TO BE A WEIGHT LOSS WINNER

You've heard the statistics. More than 90% of people who diet regain at least some weight. A National Institutes of Health panel found that people who complete weight loss programs take off about 10% of their weight, but regain two thirds of it within one year. In five years, most people regain all the lost weight, according to the NIH study.

But the news is not as dire as it sounds. Research shows us there are proven ways to stay at a healthy weight for life. In fact, thousands of people have been successful for decades at keeping unwanted pounds off.

What does it take to maintain long-term weight loss? *Have a positive attitude, perform regular vigorous exercise,* and *be mindful of what you eat.*

HOW PERSONALITY TRAITS INFLUENCE WEIGHT LOSS

Many biological traits play a role in weight loss— body size, metabolic rate, and fat and muscle content, to name a few. Personality is sometimes overlooked, but it influences our behavior in important ways. Personality traits can strengthen motivation to exercise, choose healthier foods, avoid fatty and fast foods, and limit portion sizes.

Fascinating research conducted in Japan has demonstrated that more neurotic people worry more about their health and are more willing to make sacrifices to be healthy. They also found that less agreeable people are less likely to give in to social pressure to eat.

Even more surprising were their findings on optimism. People who scored high on optimism were less likely to lose weight. It appears that being overly optimistic may cause people to underestimate their risk of developing a serious disease and think that "everything will be fine" no matter what choices they make.

Finally, they found that people who were adept at self-monitoring lost the most weight. These people were good at acquiring facts, considering options, and being objective about portion size, calories, and exercise schedules. Losing weight boosts their confidence and inspires more healthy choices and continued success.

Research conducted at Washington University School of Medicine in St. Louis, Missouri revealed that novelty-seeking or a need for adventure was associated with a higher BMI or body mass index. It appears that novelty seekers are more likely to give in to their cravings. There is no need to sit at home and suck your thumb. A better solution is for novelty seekers to seek new and different types of exercise. They can also benefit from training themselves to eat more slowly and actually savor the taste, smell, and texture of a well-prepared meal.

WEIGHT LOSS SECRETS

What are the secrets for successfully maintaining weight loss? To find out, scientists have studied people in the National Weight Control Registry (NWCR). The weight control registry was established in 1994 by James Hill, Ph.D., of the University of Colorado Health Sciences Center, and Rena Wing, Ph.D., of Brown University. Their mission was to investigate the characteristics and behaviors of people who had been successful not only at losing weight, but also keeping it off.

The registry consists of more than 3,000 people who have maintained a 30-pound weight loss for at least one year. The participants are contacted annually, and answer in-depth questionnaires about their eating and exercise habits.

"We have found four common characteristics in how people successfully keep weight off," according to Dr. Hill. "They eat a low-fat diet, weigh themselves frequently, eat breakfast every day, and engage in about 60 minutes per day of physical activity." Successful maintainers also record how much they exercise and their calorie intake, eat small meals five times a day to silence hunger pangs, and maintain consistent eating habits—that is, they tend to follow the same diet plan on weekdays and weekends.

NO QUICK FIXES

Many people don't realize that being overweight is a chronic problem. It's a condition that must be managed for life, and one that can't be resolved by going on a strict diet for a couple of months. The bad news is that there are no short-term fixes.

Making long-term lifestyle changes is the key to long-term weight loss as well as good health. Incorporating behaviors like healthy eating and daily exercise into your life—and sticking to these changes—are the framework for successfully maintaining weight loss.

FAD DIETS: NOT A SOLUTION

Fad diets are not a good strategy for maintaining weight loss in the long run.

A study published in the *New England Journal of Medicine* followed 63 obese people who were randomized to either a low-carbohydrate, high-protein diet (Atkins) or a conventional high-carbohydrate, low-fat diet. Those on the Atkins diet lost weight quickly in the first 6 months. Yet they regained much of it at the one-year mark, ending up with roughly the same amount of weight lost as those on the high-carbohydrate plan.

In both groups, cheating and dropout rates were high because the diets were not realistic for long term weight maintenance.

Studies indicate that most successful weight maintainers do not stay on fad diets or even conventional diets. Instead, they take a holistic approach to their health. They cut down on fat, and learn to snack on healthy foods—fruits, low-fat shakes, vegetables and healthy grains (whole wheat crackers or bread, for instance)—rather than junk food. They also engage in high levels of physical activity, especially strenuous activity.

According to a 13-member panel commissioned to update the Dietary Guidelines for Americans (the government's tip sheet for healthful eating), many Americans may require at least 60 minutes of physical activity most days to avoid weight gain.

The guidelines also suggest that Americans should eat a wide variety of foods, including fruits, vegetables, grains, milk products, and meat and other proteins to enable long-term weight loss.

WHAT KIND OF DIET?

In this day and age, it's easy to fall into unhealthy eating habits. High-fat foods are readily available—they're cheap, taste good, and come in super-sized portions. Studies show that eating foods low in fat as well as calories is an important factor in maintaining weight loss.

In a study published in the *Journal of the American Dietetic Association*, researchers found that a low-fat diet was instrumental for losing weight and for maintaining weight loss.

They followed 38 overweight women who participated in a 26-week weight-loss program. While on the program, the women adhered to a very-low-calorie diet and lost an average of 46 pounds each. Three years after the program ended, researchers were able to contact 27 of the original 38 women. The women gained back an average of 71.5% of the weight they had lost—but some subjects regained less than 2% of their initial weight loss.

How did they do it? Those who kept their fat intake to 25% or less of calories per day and were more active regained less weight.

HEALTHY DIETING IS EASIER

Compared to fad diets, well-balanced eating is actually easier. There are several ways to maintain a healthy diet, and choosing the best and easiest strategy for you is important.

Here are some tips:

- Eat a lot of fish, vegetables, and chicken.
- Limit fried foods.
- Drink a glass of water 15 minutes before meals.

CHAPTER II

- Have a clear based soup before dinner.
- At a restaurant, order an appetizer, rather than a whole entrée.
- Grill foods to reduce fat.
- To enhance taste of healthy foods, use fresh herbs. You can grow them in your garden.
- Practice portion control. That's especially important at restaurants, where diners are often served huge entrees—as much as two to five times the size of a normal serving. To cut down on overeating at restaurants, aim to eat only half your entrée, and put the rest in the doggie bag when the entreé is served.
- Eat slowly to cut down on overeating. It takes the hypothalamus at least 20 minutes to realize you're full, courtesy of CCK and PPY release from the duodenum.

MOM WAS RIGHT: EAT YOUR BREAKFAST

People who maintain their weight over the long-term share one important habit: *eating breakfast*. In fact, 78% of the participants in the NWCR say they eat breakfast every day of the week. Very few of the successful weight-loss maintainers report never eating breakfast.

According to a study published in *Obesity Research*, eating breakfast may stave off hunger that appears later in the day—hunger that may lead to over-eating. Researchers have also found that breakfast eaters chose less energy-dense foods (with fewer calories) during the remainder of the day, and are more likely to be

eating breakfast may stave off hunger that appears later in the day.

physically active. People who eat breakfast every day, on average, consume 200 calories less than those who skip breakfast.

There are many low-fat and low-calorie breakfast choices available. A meal of eggs with whole-wheat toast is a healthy breakfast, but try your toast with jelly or fat-free spread. Oatmeal and whole grain cereal with skim milk is high in fiber and low in calories. A piece of fruit on the side can add variety, or you can make a fresh fruit salad with granola on top for some crunch.

Quick Tips
How to Eat Forbidden Foods

You can eat forbidden foods—chocolate and cheesecake—and still maintain your weight. Just spend your calories wisely. Here are some other ways to enjoy high-calorie foods without the worry:

• Eat smaller portions

• Split dessert with a friend

• Order any sauces or dressings on the side

• Choose a low-fat version

• Purchase single serving portions and cut them in half

• Choose a snack-size candy bar—the size you give kids at Halloween

• Indulge your sweet tooth each day with a small amount of high quality chocolate. Many people find dark chocolate the most satisfying, and it contains antioxidants.

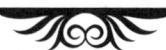

GET SOME EXPERT ADVICE

Working with an experienced dietitian or nutritionist may also help you eat more healthfully in the long run. A two-year study published in the *Journal of the American Dietetic Association* found that women who work with diet professionals to develop lowfat eating plans have more success than women who monitor their own eating habits without the support of a diet professional.

In this study, 12,000 postmenopausal women were enrolled in a nutritionist-directed program aimed at reducing fat intake to 20% of total calories, or devised their own eating plan. The women who worked with nutritionists attended regular group support meetings. There the nutritionists emphasized behavioral skills, self-reliance, social support, and methods to prevent relapse. By the end of the study's first year, women who had worked with a professional reduced their total fat intake from 38.5% of calories to 24.3%. Women in the study who hadn't gone through any intervention were consuming 35.7% of calories from fat.

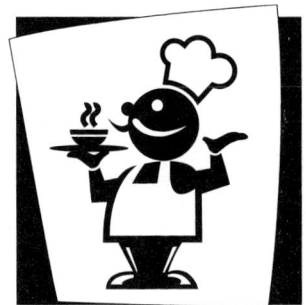

By the end of the second year, women with professional support recorded 25.4% fat intake, while the other women recorded 36% fat intake.

Studies tell us that people who keep track of their progress are more likely to maintain weight loss. That often means noting down your weight, food intake, and amount of exercise each day in a journal.

You can also keep track of the moods that cause you to overeat, as well as what foods tempt you to overindulge. This type of record-keeping takes some effort, but it can help identify your "triggers" for overeating.

Keeping tabs on your diet progress—called "self-monitoring"—reinforces your commitment to change while increasing your feeling of control. Self-monitoring can improve mood and provide a sense of self-efficacy, as well as clarifying eating and exercise patterns.

MOTIVATION COUNTS

Many people become more successful at long-term weight loss *when their motive changes from wanting to be skinnier to wanting to be healthier.* The right attitude means everything when it comes to keeping weight off. It's important to stay focused

Quick Tips: Easy Ways to Change Bad Habits

Here are some minor changes you can make in your eating habits—they'll help you cut calories, eat healthier, and maintain your weight.

- Coffeehouse drinks are often big on calories, because they're often laden with chocolate, whole milk and whipped cream. To slim down on these drinks, ask for fat-free milk with no whipped cream, chocolate sprinkles or syrup

- To reduce the fat in ground beef, brown it, then put it in a colander and bathe it with boiling water

- On salads, use crumbled-up flavored rice cakes rather than oily croutons

- Cut back on sodas and fruit juice—they're high in calories. Instead dilute your fruit juice or soda with lots of ice or club soda. Or better yet, substitute foods that are really good for you: Real fruit and water

- Always measure the oil you cook with or use on salads. It's easy to misjudge the amount you "drizzle" on a salad or into the frying pan. A quarter cup of oil can add almost 500 calories to your diet

- If you don't like to count calories, try this method of eating healthier. Fill half your plate with vegetables and fruits. Divide the other half exactly between meat and starch.

- Experiment with a meatless menu a few days a week to see if you enjoy it. Stir-fried tofu, soy burgers, and vegetable stews can all be made into delicious and low-fat entrees. (But a word to the wise: when eating vegetarian, choose low-fat milk, cheese and yogurt.)

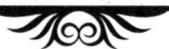

on the positives and realize there will be setbacks, but that it's possible to recover from them.

Let's face it, life happens. We get new jobs, lose a job, fall in love, fall out of love, get sick, and see a loved one become seriously ill. Our lives are constantly changing. That's why we need to consciously and constantly monitor the way we live, and the impact of life events on our eating and exercise habits.

A study published in the *American Journal of Clinical Nutrition* found that attitude can significantly affect weight loss maintenance. In the study, researchers evaluated the behavioral characteristics of those who successfully maintained weight loss over two years.

The researchers followed 714 NWCR participants who had lost an average of 64 pounds. After following them for two years, the researchers discovered that 66% of participants regained weight after one year. Of those, only 11% were able to return to their initial weight.

However, over 99% of participants remained at or below their recommended lifetime weight.

Those who regained weight and then failed to take off the added pounds were more likely to have symptoms of depression. Previous studies have found that people who suffer from depression or those who more frequently experience "the blues," are more likely to overeat, less likely to exercise and tend to regain pounds after losing weight.

FIND A WEIGHT LOSS BUDDY

Only you can lose weight and keep it off, but it sure is nice to know your friends and family are behind you all the way.

Becoming discouraged is often the biggest obstacle to maintaining weight loss. Support from a friend, family member, formal support group, or even an Internet-based group can help you stay motivated and on track. Studies show that people who participate in weight loss treatment with a friend or family member do better than those without a supportive buddy.

At work, ask coworkers if they'd like to go for a brisk walk during lunch. Call or email long-distance friends to stay in touch and share your weight loss progress. Form your own mini-support group.

Joining a formal support group can also work. Howard Rankin, Ph.D., is a psychologist at TOPS (Take Off Pounds Sensibly). In the TOPS program, people are free to follow any diet plan, but meet every week in a support group. According to Dr. Rankin, support groups are often a place where struggling dieters can find encouragement for adhering to their weight loss programs. Support groups can work by keeping dieters accountable, providing inspiration, and serving as a forum where dieters can share information and tips for losing weight.

DO INTERNET SUPPORT GROUPS WORK?

In an age of wireless Internet devices and smartphones, many people are taking advantage of online support groups and online therapists. Internet groups can help people lose weight, according to recent studies. The convenience of the Internet means that one can find support at any time, anywhere.

Internet support is a good option for those people who are busy, who live in remote locations, or can't afford to attend support group meetings.

There is evidence that Internet support groups may be just as effective as face-to-face meetings for support. In one study published in *Obesity Research*, 255 people participated in a six-month weight control program conducted over interactive television, followed by a one-year maintenance program.

During that year, participants were split into three groups; the first, with frequent in-person support; the second, with minimal in-person support; and the third, with Internet support, including online chat groups.

The result? Researchers found that participants assigned to the Internet-based weight maintenance program kept off as much weight as those who continued to meet face-to-face.

MAKE EXERCISE PART OF YOUR LIFESTYLE

People who are successful at maintaining weight loss share a common characteristic: a dedication to an active lifestyle. Exercise is not only good for your body; it makes you feel good too. Increasing your activity level burns calories, and is just as vital for maintaining weight as for weight loss.

Unfortunately, most people lose weight through cutting calories, and don't increase physical activity. Weight maintainers in the NWCR report that, on average, they burn off around 400 calories a day through exercise—about the equivalent of a brisk 60 to 75 minute walk.

The American College of Sports Medicine recommends at least 30 minutes of aerobic activity five days a week. Without exercise, the average person gains a pound a year between ages 25 and 55. Those who are already overweight tend to gain more per year.

To get the benefits of exercise, it's not necessary to join a gym. It doesn't matter how you stay active, as long as you find a way to exercise regularly. While walking is by far the most common form of exercise, anything that increases your activity level counts—gardening, housework, yard work, cleaning, or decorating. Take a dance class, climb the stairs at work, or keep hand weights near the TV and pump some iron during

Quick Tips

Good Ways to Keep Track

- Keep a journal. By assessing your progress in a journal, you can evaluate whether you are sticking to your weight maintenance goals, or if you're headed for weight regain. Pin down the places where you tend to overeat, and when you're most likely to snack. Then you can modify your behaviors.

- Keeping a food journal can be as simple as writing down meals in a notebook or on the computer. Day-by-day bound food and exercise journals are sold in stationery stores or you can try 3" x 5" index cards.

- Weigh yourself twice a week, and measure your waistline every few weeks. Then keep track of the changes. It will keep you motivated to stay on a healthy diet.

your favorite shows. FitBit type tracking devices are helpful for many people.

It's easy to get hooked on exercise because of the feel-good endorphins and positive feelings that come with it. Pick an activity or exercise you enjoy and make it a priority. Start with setting a goal. The longer you exercise and the more often you exercise, the more calories you burn.

CHAPTER 11

Weight maintenance isn't easy. About one third of the NWCR participants describe weight maintenance as difficult, one third as moderately easy, and one third as easy. No matter how frustrated you get, stay focused on your goals. No one is perfect. You're likely to have an occasional setback and gain a few pounds. Instead of giving up, simply start fresh.

One study of people who were successful at weight loss, published in the *Journal of Consulting and Clinical Psychology*, looked at why people backslide after weight loss. The researchers found that risk factors for regaining weight include: a more recent weight loss (less than two years versus more than two years), a weight loss of 30% of body weight or more, and binge eating.

The people who regained weight reported that they decreased their activity levels after the initial weight loss and increased the percentage of calories from fat. They also said they felt hungrier and felt less restraint when it came to eating unhealthy foods.

The study authors suggest that several years of successful weight maintenance increases your chance of keeping the weight off. It also helps you continue behavioral lifestyle changes that helped you lose weight initially.

One of the best strategies to prevent backsliding is to record your weight weekly, and graph your progress. Minor fluctuations in weight are to be expected during the weight loss and maintenance process. By graphing your weight you can learn to anticipate temporary setbacks. The graph lines may bounce up and down like a seismograph recording during an earthquake, but there should be an overall downward trend.

Successful weight maintainers who weigh themselves regularly are able to recognize weight gain early—and able to get back on track right away. Keeping close watch on their weight helps them to identify even a small weight gain and to make appropriate behavioral adjustments.

When you notice a red flag like a steady increase in weight, acknowledge the trend as a minor setback, but don't comfort yourself by heading for the ice cream store or lapsing into eating high calorie, high fat meals. Think positive and forgive yourself. Do the best you can every day and reaffirm your commitment to a healthy lifestyle.

To get back on track after a weight gain, start immediately. Go for a short brisk walk or plan some healthy meals for the remainder of the day. Gradually increase the duration and intensity of your workouts, keep a close eye on your portion size, and drink more water. If you're bored with your routine, add a new activity that you've never tried before—maybe join a yoga class or softball team, or sign up for ballroom dancing and actually go! Keep in mind that it's important to stick with the methods that work best for you.

Empower yourself by focusing on what you can impact—your behavior—instead of the numbers on the scale. Backsliding happens to everyone, and you should view it as an opportunity to learn from your mistakes.

SET REALISTIC GOALS

Losing weight and keeping pounds off is a lifelong journey. Whether you lose weight on your own or with a group, remember that the most important changes are gradual and long-term. No matter how much weight you have lost, modest goals and a commitment to a healthy lifestyle will increase your chances of keeping it off.

Goals should be reasonable and realistic, so that you have a good chance of achieving them. It is realistic to lose a pound or two a week and to exercise three times per week. If you have high expectations—for example, you aim to lose 5 pounds a week—then you are likely to get frustrated and give up. Unrealistic weight goals cause many people to fail. You didn't gain weight overnight and, consequently, you shouldn't expect to lose weight overnight either. Be patient and work toward your goal day by day. Once you meet your goal, you can always reevaluate and create new ones.

WHAT I DO (REALLY)

I'm 64. Over the past 40 years I've cared for patients in a private practice, taught medical students, residents, and fellows in hospitals, traveled across the country lecturing, and spent endless hours writing and editing. For nearly 7 years I took care of sick, elderly parents, and in recent years, I've been sidelined by a frustrating number of autoimmune disorders. I have given in to the temptation to stuff my face with M&M's at 3 a.m. in airports and hospital rooms. None of that is conducive to having a slender body. But if you don't practice what you preach most of the time, people will spot it in a heartbeat. So research findings aside, here's a thumbnail sketch of what I really do to stay slender.

- ᔆ Eat breakfast everyday. I alternate between oatmeal or another whole grain cereal with a one-egg omelette. The yolk is fine. It's a good source of choline (think acetylcholine, the neurotransmitter that's crucial for memory). The cereal is just enough to fill a small custard cup. I use 1% milk and sometimes a few blueberries with a cup of tea. No sugar.

- ᔆ I make sandwiches with one slice of oatmeal or whole-grain bread.

- ᔆ Everything I serve myself is on a little salad plate or luncheon plate. No full-size dinner plates for me.

- ᔆ Never eat anything right out of the bag, box, can, or container, even if no one is looking.

Take a handful of nuts, dried fruit, animal crackers, or even chocolate chips on a little dish, and eat one at a time—slowly.

∾ Never waste calories on anything that isn't fabulous.

∾ Try not to drink too many calories. Water really is best most of the time.

∾ Order from the children's menu if all else fails.

∾ Never eat until you feel full. Slow down enough to recognize when the sensation of hunger abates. Small amounts of food every few hours makes it easier to stay energetic.

∾ Eat a little bit of whole-grain cereal an hour or so before bedtime.

∾ Keep *Boost* or *Carnation Breakfast Essentials* handy for times when I'm feeling depleted and hungry, but stressed, and in a hurry. Yes, they contain some sugar, but it's better than heading for a 600-calorie mocha-cocoa-loco latte somewhere.

∾ Travel with my own snacks—breakfast bars, peppermint patties (lowfat and refreshing), ziplock baggies with nuts or cereal. I'm too ill to travel now, but this worked for years.

ᴄᴠ Take the stairs whenever I can.

ᴄᴠ Alternate walking with a Pilates routine every other day.

ᴄᴠ Do my own pruning, trimming, and weeding in the yard. It gives my neighbors something to watch.

ᴄᴠ Do my own housework—if I hired a maid, I'd just clean the house before she came over anyway.

THE BOTTOM LINE: WEIGHT LOSS THAT WORKS

It doesn't matter what "diet" you use. I've never been an advocate of "dieting." Consider the first three letters of the word. The real key to maintaining your weight loss is to make a commitment to a healthy lifestyle. The only way to lose weight and keep it off is to burn more calories than you consume regularly.

The trick is to find a way to maintain weight loss that works for you—whether it is through ballet classes, a food diary, a weekly Internet support group, or even something as simple as a morning walk through the neighborhood. This chapter has given you several tools to use in your arsenal against weight gain, but it all comes down to you. Create a plan to fit your life that includes regular exercise and eating less fat, less sugar, fewer calories, and more vegetables and fruits.

Once you view weight maintenance in terms of being healthy instead of being skinny, you'll be taking steps toward a lifelong lifestyle change.

Remember, it's not about fitting into a size six dress, achieving an ideal figure, or dropping a certain number of pounds. It's about reaching a healthy weight—one that makes you feel good about yourself—and maintaining that weight loss for life. If you succeed, you'll not only be healthier and more fit, but you'll probably live a longer, more enjoyable life. Perhaps, along the way, you'll be able to help a few other folks do the same.

REFERENCES

1. Academy of Nutrition and Dietetics. Tips for Weight Loss. How to Handle Food Cravings. https://www.eatright.org/health/weight-loss/tips-for-weight-loss

2. Adams, T.D., Davidson, L.E., Litwin, S.E., et al. (2017). Weight and metabolic outcomes 12 years after gastric bypass. *New England Journal of Medicine,* 377(12), 1143-1155. DOI: 10.1056/NEJMoa1700459

3. Agnoli, C., Sieri, S., Ricceri, F., et al. (2018). Adherence to a Mediterranean diet and long-term changes in weight and waist circumference in the EPIC-Italy cohort. *Nutrition & Diabetes,* 8(1), 22. DOI: 10.1038/s41387-018-0023-3

4. Anton, S.D., Hida, A., Heekin, K., et al. (2017). Effects of Popular Diets without Specific Calorie Targets on Weight Loss Outcomes: Systematic Review of Findings from Clinical Trials. *Nutrients,* 9(8), pii: E822. DOI: 10.3390/nu9080822

5. Aragon, A.A., Schoenfeld, B.J., Wildman, R., et al. (2017). International society of sports nutrition position stand: diets and body composition. *Journal of the International Society for Sports Nutrition,* 14, 16. DOI: 10.1186/s12970-017-0174-y

6. Arthritis Foundation. How Fat Affects Arthritis. https://www.arthritis.org/living-with-arthritis/comorbidities/obesity-arthritis/fat-and-arthritis.php

7. Barnes, A.S. (2013). Emerging modifiable risk factors for cardiovascular disease in women: obesity, physical activity, and sedentary behavior. *Texas Heart Institute Journal,* 40(3), 293-295.

8. Barnes, A.S., (2011). The Epidemic of Obesity and Diabetes. Trends and Treatments. *Texas Heart Institute Journal,* 38(2), 142–144.

9. Barnett, T.A., Kelly, A.S., Young, D.R., et al. (2018). Sedentary Behaviors in Today's Youth: Approaches to the Prevention and Management of Childhood Obesity: A Scientific Statement From the American Heart Association. *Circulation,* 138(11), e142-e159. DOI: 10.1161/CIR.0000000000000591

10. Bayon, V., Leger, D., Gomez-Merino, D, et al. (2014). Sleep debt and obesity. *Annals of Medicine,* 46(5), 264-272. DOI: 10.3109/07853890.2014.931103.

11. Bazan, I.S., Fares, W.H. (2016). Review of the Ongoing Story of Appetite Suppressants, Serotonin Pathway, and Pulmonary Vascular Disease. *American Journal of Cardiology*, 117(10), 1691-1696. DOI: 10.1016/j.amjcard.2016.02.049

12. Beccuti, G., Pannain, S. (2011). Sleep and obesity. *Current Opinion in Clinical Nutrition & Metabolic Care*, 14(4), 402–412. DOI: 10.1097/MCO.0b013e3283479109

13. Beck, C., Fausett, J.K., Krukowski, R.A., et al. (2013). A randomized trial of a community-based cognitive intervention for obese senior adults. *Journal of Aging and Health*, 25(1), 97-118. DOI: 10.1177/0898264312467374

14. Better Health Channel/Jean Hailes for Women's Health. (2018). Menopause and Weight Gain. https://www.betterhealth.vic.gov.au/health/ConditionsAndTreatments/menopause-and-weight-gain?viewAsPdf=true

15. Bhat, S.P., Sharma, A. (2017). Current Drug Targets in Obesity Pharmacotherapy - A Review. *Current Drug Targets*, 18(8), 983-993. DOI: 10.2174/1389450118666170227153940

16. Blau, L.E., Orloff, N.C., Flammer, A., et al. (2018). Food craving frequency mediates the relationship between emotional eating and excess weight gain in pregnancy. *Eating Behaviors*, 31, 120-124. DOI: 10.1016/j.eatbeh.2018.09.004

17. Bohula, E.A., Wiviott, S.D., Mcguire, D.K., et al. (2018). Cardiovascular safety of lorcaserin in overweight or obese patients. *New England Journal of Medicine*, 379(12), 1107-1111. DOI: 10.1056/NEJMoa1808721

18. Boswell, R.G., Kober, H. (2016). Food cue reactivity and craving predict eating and weight gain: a meta-analytic review. *Obesity Reviews*, 17(2), 159-177. DOI: 10.1111/obr.12354

19. Broughton, D.E., Moley, K.H. (2017). Obesity and female infertility: potential mediators of obesity's impact. *Fertility and Sterility*, 107(4), 840-847. DOI: 10.1016/j.fertnstert.2017.01.017

20. Bueno, N.B., de Melo, I.S., de Oliveira, S.L., da Rocha, Ataide, T. (2013). Very-low-carbohydrate ketogenic diet v. low-fat diet for long-term weight loss: a meta-analysis of randomised controlled trials. *British Journal of Nutrition*, 110(7), 1178-1187. DOI: 10.1017/S0007114513000548

21. Centers for Disease Control and Prevention. (2018). Adult Obesity Causes & Consequences. https://www.cdc.gov/obesity/adult/causes.html

22. Centers for Disease Control and Prevention. (2018). Adult Obesity Facts. https://www.cdc.gov/obesity/data/adult.html

23. Centers for Disease Control and Prevention. (2013). Asthma and Obesity. https://www.cdc.gov/asthma/asthma_stats/asthma_obesity.htm

24. Centers for Disease Control and Prevention. (2018). Myalgic Encephalomyelitis/Chronic Fatigue Syndrome. https://www.cdc.gov/me-cfs/

25. Centers for Disease Control and Prevention. Public Health Genomics. (2011). Obesity and Genetics: What We Know, What We Don't Know and What it Means. https://www.cdc.gov/genomics/resources/diseases/obesity/obesknow.htm

26. Chen, C.C., Liu, K., Hsu, C.C., et al. (2017). Healthy lifestyle and normal waist circumference are associated with a lower 5-year risk of type 2 diabetes in middle-aged and elderly individuals: Results from the healthy aging longitudinal study in Taiwan (HALST). *Medicine (Baltimore)*, 96(6), e6025. DOI: 10.1097/MD.0000000000006025.

27. Churuangsuk, C., Kherouf, M., Combet, E., Lean M. (2018). Low-carbohydrate diets for overweight and obesity: a systematic review of the systematic reviews. *Obesity Reviews*, Sep 7. DOI: 10.1111/obr.12744

28. Collet, T.H., van der Klaauw, A.A., Henning, E., et al. (2016). The Sleep/Wake Cycle is Directly Modulated by Changes in Energy Balance. *Sleep*, 39(9), 1691-700. DOI: 10.5665/sleep.6094

29. Colquitt, J.L., Pickett. K., Loveman, E., Frampton, G.K. (2014). Surgery for weight loss in adults. *The Cochrane Database of Systematic Reviews*, (8):CD003641. DOI: 10.1002/14651858.CD003641.pub4

30. Conway, B.N., Han, X., Munro, H.M., et al. (2018). The obesity epidemic and rising diabetes incidence in a low-income racially diverse southern US cohort. *PLoS One*,13(1), e0190993. DOI: 10.1371/journal.pone.0190993.

31. Coulter, A.A., Rebello, C.J., Greenway, F.L. (2018). Centrally Acting Agents for Obesity: Past, Present, and Future. *Drugs*, 78(11), 1113-1132. DOI: 10.1007/s40265-018-0946-y

32. Crönlein, T. (2016). Insomnia and obesity. *Current Opinion in Psychiatry*, 29(6), 409-412. doi: 10.1097/YCO.0000000000000284

33. Di Daniele, N., Noce, A., Vidiri, M.F., et al. (2017). Impact of Mediterranean diet on metabolic syndrome, cancer and longevity. *Oncotarget,* 8(5), 8947-8979. DOI: 10.18632/oncotarget.13553.

34. de Carvalho, M.M.B., Coutinho, R.Q., Barros, I.M.L., et al. (2018). Prevalence of Obstructive Sleep Apnea and Obesity Among Middle-Aged Women: Implications for Exercise Capacity. *Journal of Clinical Sleep Medicine,* 14(9), 1471-1475. DOI: 10.5664/jcsm.7316

35. de Oliveira Otto, M.C., Anderson, C.A.M., Dearborn, J.L., et al; American Heart Association Behavioral Change for Improving Health Factors Committee of the Council on Lifestyle and Cardiometabolic Health and Council on Epidemiology and Prevention; Council on Cardiovascular and Stroke Nursing; Council on Clinical Cardiology; and Stroke Council. (2018). Dietary Diversity: Implications for Obesity Prevention in Adult Populations: A Science Advisory From the American Heart Association. *Circulation,*138(11), e160-e168. DOI: 10.1161/CIR.0000000000000595

36. de Rooij, B.H., van der Berg, J.D., van der Kallen, C.J., et al. (2016). Physical Activity and Sedentary Behavior in Metabolically Healthy versus Unhealthy Obese and Non-Obese Individuals - The Maastricht Study. *PLoS One,* 3;11(5), e0154358. DOI: 10.1371/journal.pone.0154358

37. Devonport, T.J., Nicholls, W., Fullerton, C. (2017). A systematic review of the association between emotions and eating behaviour in normal and overweight adult populations. *Journal of Health Psychology,* 7 Mar 1:1359105317697813. DOI: 10.1177/1359105317697813Diet, drugs, devices and surgery for weight management. (2018). *The Medical Letter on Drugs and Therapeutics,* 60(1548), 91-94.

38. Diet, drugs, and surgery for weight loss. (2011). *Treatment Guidelines from The Medical Letter,* 9(104), 17-22.

39. Di Germanio, C., Di Francesco, A., Bernier, M., de Cabo, R. (2018). Yo-Yo Dieting is Better than None. *Obesity (Silver Spring),* 26(11), 1673. DOI: 10.1002/oby.22335

40. Drugs for Type 2 Diabetes. (2011). *Treatment Guidelines from The Medical Letter,* 9(108), 47-54.

41. Eckel, R.H., Kahn, S.E., Ferannini, E., et al. (2011). Obesity and Type 2 Diabetes: What Can Be Unified and What Needs to Be Individualized? Consensus Statement. *The Journal of Clinical Endocrinology & Management,* 96(6), 1654–1663. DOI: 10.1210/jc.2011-0585

42. Esposito, K., Kastorini, C.M., Panagiotakos, D.B., Giugliano, D. (2011). Mediterranean diet and weight loss: meta-analysis of randomized controlled trials. *Metabolic Syndrome and Related Disorders*, 9(1), 1-12. DOI: 10.1089/met.2010.0031

43. Evers, C., Dingemans, A., Junghans, A.F, Boevé, A. (2018). Feeling bad or feeling good, does emotion affect your consumption of food? A meta-analysis of the experimental evidence. *Neuroscience and Biobehavioral Reviews*, 92, 195-208. DOI: 10.1016/j.neubiorev.2018.05.028

44. Farpour-Lambert, N.J., Ells, L.J., Martinez de Tejada, B., Scott, C. (2018). Obesity and Weight Gain in Pregnancy and Postpartum: an Evidence Review of Lifestyle Interventions to Inform Maternal and Child Health Policies. *Frontiers in Endocrinology (Lausanne)*, 9, 546. DOI: 10.3389/fendo.2018.00546

45. Flores, S., Brown, A., Adeoye, S., et al. (2013). Examining the impact of obesity on individuals with chronic fatigue syndrome. *Workplace Health & Safety*, 61(7), 299-307. DOI: 10.3928/21650799-20130617-12

46. Forno, E., Celedón, J.C. (2017). The effect of obesity, weight gain, and weight loss on asthma inception and control. *Current Opinion in Allergy and Clinical Immunology*, 17(2), 123-130. DOI: 10.1097/ACI.0000000000000339

47. Frasca, D., Blomberg, B.B., Paganelli, R. (2017). Aging, Obesity, and Inflammatory Age-Related Diseases. *Frontiers in Immunology*, 8, 1745. DOI: 10.3389/fimmu.2017.01745

48. Frayn, M., Livshits, S., Knäuper, B. (2018). Emotional eating and weight regulation: a qualitative study of compensatory behaviors and concerns. *Journal of Eating Disorders*, 6, 23. DOI: 10.1186/s40337-018-0210-6

49. Fruh, S.M. (2017). Obesity: Risk factors, complications, and strategies for sustainable long-term weight management. *Journal of the American Association of Nurse Practitioners*, 29(S1), S3-S14. DOI: 10.1002/2327-6924.12510

50. Gambero, A., Ribeiro, M.L. (2015). The positive effects of yerba maté (Ilex paraguariensis) in obesity. *Nutrients*, 7(2), 730-750. DOI: 10.3390/nu7020730

51. Gardner, C.D., Kiazand, A., Alhassan, S., et al. (2007). Comparison of the Atkins, Zone, Ornish, and LEARN diets for change in weight and related risk factors among overweight premenopausal women: the A TO Z Weight Loss Study: a randomized trial. *Journal of the American Medical Association*, 297(9), 969-977.

52. Garg SK, Maurer H, Reed K, Selagamsetty R. (2014). Diabetes and cancer: two diseases with obesity as a common risk factor. *Diabetes, Obesity & Metabolism*, 16(2), 97-110. DOI: 10.1111/dom.12124

53. The GBD 2015 Obesity Collaborators. (2017). Health effects of overweight and obesity in 195 countries over 25 years. *New England Journal of Medicine*, 377(1), 13-27. DOI: 10.1056/NEJMoa1614362

54. Gibson, A.A., Seimon, R.V., Lee, C.M., et al. (2015). Do ketogenic diets really suppress appetite? A systematic review and meta-analysis. *Obesity Reviews*, 16(1), 64-76. DOI: 10.1111/obr.12230

55. Greydanus, D.E., Agana, M., Kamboj, M.K., et al. (2018). Pediatric obesity: Current concepts. *Disease-a-Month: DM*, 64(4), 98-156. DOI: 10.1016/j.disamonth.2017.12.001

56. Ha, H., Han, D., Kim. B. (2017). Can Obesity Cause Depression? A Pseudo-panel Analysis. *Journal of Preventive Medicine and Public Health*. 50(4), 262–267. DOI: 10.3961/jpmph.17.067

57. Heriseanu, A.I., Hay, P., Corbit, L., Touyz, S. (2017). Grazing in adults with obesity and eating disorders: A systematic review of associated clinical features and meta-analysis of prevalence. *Clinical Psychology Review*, 58, 16-32. DOI: 10.1016/j.cpr.2017.09.004

58. Hickner, J. (2016). Is the Rx to blame for the patient's weight gain? *Journal of Family Practice*, 65(11), 753.Hofmann, W., Friese, M. (2011). Control Yourself! How to Keep Cravings in Check. *Scientific American Mind*, May/June, 43-47.

59. Hill, A.J., Cairnduff, V., McCance, D.R. (2016). Nutritional and clinical associations of food cravings in pregnancy. *Journal of Human Nutrition and Dietetics*, 29(3), 281-289. DOI: 10.1111/jhn.12333

60. Hochberg. Z. (2018). An Evolutionary Perspective on the Obesity Epidemic. *Trends in Endocrinology and Metabolism: TEM*. pii: S1043-2760(18)30163-2. DOI: 10.1016/j.tem.2018.09.002

61. Hormes, J.M., Niemiec, M.A. (2017). Does culture create craving? Evidence from the case of menstrual chocolate craving. *PLoS One*, 12(7), e0181445. DOI: 10.1371/journal.pone.0181445

62. Hormes, J.M., Orloff, N.C., Timko, C.A. (2014). Chocolate craving and disordered eating. Beyond the gender divide? *Appetite*, 83, 185-193. DOI: 10.1016/j.appet.2014.08.018

63. Ikramuddin, S., Blackstone, R.P., Brancatisano, A., et al. (2014). Effect of reversible intermittent intra-abdominal vagal nerve blockade on morbid obesity: the ReCharge randomized clinical trial. *Journal of the American Medical Association*, 312(9), 915-922. DOI: 10.1001/jama.2014.10540

64. Jabr, F. (2017). Why exercise may be the best fix for depression. *Scientific American Mind*, 28(1):27-31.

65. James, W.P.T., Caterson, I.D., Coutinho, W., et al. (2010). Effect of Sibutramine on cardiovascular outcomes in overweight and obese subjects. *New England Journal of Medicine*, 363(10), 905-917. DOI: 10.1056/NEJMoa1003114

66. Jantaratnotai, N., Mosikanon, K., Lee, Y., McIntyre, R.S. (2017). The interface of depression and obesity. *Obesity Research & Clinical Practice*, 11(1), 1-10. DOI: 10.1016/j.orcp.2016.07.003

67. Johnston, B.C, Kanters, S., Bandayrel, K., et al. (2014). Comparison of weight loss among named diet programs in overweight and obese adults: a meta-analysis. *Journal of the American Medical Association*, 312(9), 923-933. DOI: 10.1001/jama.2014.10397

68. Joyner, M.A., Gearhardt, A.N., White, M.A. (2015). Food craving as a mediator between addictive-like eating and problematic eating outcomes. *Eating Behaviors*, 19, 98-101. DOI: 10.1016/j.eatbeh.2015.07.005

69. Jungheim, E.S., Travieso, J.L., Carson, K.R., Moley, K.H. (2012). Obesity and Reproductive Function. *Obstetrics and Gynecology Clinics of North America*, 39(4), 479–493. DOI: 10.1016/j.ogc.2012.09.002

70. Kahan, S. (2017). Obesity and sleep: an evolving relationship. *Sleep Health*, 3(5), 381-382. DOI: 10.1016/j.sleh.2017.07.010

71. Katterman, S.N., Kleinman, B.M., Hood, M.M., et al. (2014). Mindfulness meditation as an intervention for binge eating, emotional eating, and weight loss: a systematic review. *Eating Behaviors*, 15(2), 197-204. DOI: 10.1016/j.eatbeh.2014.01.005

72. Khera, R., Murad, M.H., Chandar, A.K., et al. (2016). Association of Pharmacological Treatments for Obesity With Weight Loss and Adverse Events: A Systematic Review and Meta-analysis. *Journal of the American Medical Association*, 315(22), 2424-2434. DOI: 10.1001/jama.2016.7602

73. King., K.K., March, L., Anandacoomarasamy, A. (2013). Obesity & osteoarthritis. *Indian Journal of Medical Research*, 138(2), 185–193.

74. Kobayashi, D., Takahashi, O., Deshpande, G.A, et al. (2012). Association between weight gain, obesity, and sleep duration: a large-scale 3-year cohort study. *Sleep and Breathing*, 16(3), 829-833. DOI: 10.1007/s11325-011-0583-0

75. Koliaki, C., Spinos, T., Spinou, M., et al. (2018). Defining the Optimal Dietary Approach for Safe, Effective and Sustainable Weight Loss in Overweight and Obese Adults. *Healthcare (Basel)*, 6(3), pii: E73. DOI: 10.3390/healthcare6030073

76. Lavie, C.J., Laddu. D., Arena, R., et al. (2018). Healthy Weight and Obesity Prevention: JACC Health Promotion Series. *Journal of the American College of Cardiology*, 72(13), 1506-1531. DOI: 10.1016/j.jacc.2018.08.1037

77. Lavie, C.J., Milani, R.V., Artham, S.M., et al (2009). The obesity paradox, weight loss, and coronary disease. *American Journal of Medicine* 122(12), 1106-1114. DOI: 10.1016/j.amjmed.2009.06.006

78. Lim, S.S., Davies, M.J., Norman, R.J., Moran, L.J. (2012). Overweight, obesity and central obesity in women with polycystic ovary syndrome: a systematic review and meta-analysis. *Human Reproduction Update*, 18(6), 618-637. DOI: 10.1093/humupd/dms030

79. Lim, S.S., Norman, R.J., Davies, M.J., Moran, L.J. (2013). The effect of obesity on polycystic ovary syndrome: a systematic review and meta-analysis. *Obesity Reviews*, 14(2), 95-109. DOI: 10.1111/j.1467-789X.2012.01053.x

80. Liu, Z., Zhang, T.T., Yu, J., et al. (2016). Excess Body Weight during Childhood and Adolescence Is Associated with the Risk of Multiple Sclerosis: A Meta-Analysis. *Neuroepidemiology*, 47(2), 103-108.

81. Ludwig, D.S., Ebbeling, C.B. (2018). The Carbohydrate-Insulin Model of Obesity: Beyond "Calories In, Calories Out". *JAMA Internal Medicine*, 178(8), 1098-1103. DOI: 10.1001/jamainternmed.2018.2933

82. Mantzios, M., Wilson, J.C. (2015). Mindfulness, Eating Behaviours, and Obesity: A Review and Reflection on Current Findings. *Current Obesity Reports*, 4(1), 141-146. DOI: 10.1007/s13679-014-0131-x

83. Mateo-Gallego, R., Marco-Benedí ,V.2, Perez-Calahorra, S., et al. (2017). Energy-restricted, high-protein diets more effectively impact cardiometabolic profile in overweight and obese women than lower-protein diets. *Clinical Nutrition*, 36(2), 371-379. DOI: 10.1016/j.clnu.2016.01.018

84. Medline Plus. Medical Encyclopedia. Pseudohypoparathyroidism. www.nlm.nih.gov/medlineplus/ency/article/000364.htm.

85. Medscape. (2018). Anxiety Disorders. https://emedicine. medscape.com/article/286227-overview

86. Mehaffey, J.H., LaPar, D.J., Clement, K.C., et al. (2016). 10 year outcomes after roux-en-Y gastric bypass. *Annals of Surgery,* 264(1), 121-126. DOI: 10.1097/SLA.0000000000001544

87. *The Merck Manual,* 20th Edition. Chapter 239. Sleep and Wakefulness Disorders. pp. 2013-2026. Merck and Co., Inc. 2018.

88. Minkwitz, J., Scheipl, F., Cartwright, L., et al. (2018). Why some obese people become depressed whilst others do not: exploring links between cognitive reactivity, depression and obesity. *Psychology, Health & Medicine,* Sep 25, 1-12. DOI: 10.1080/13548506.2018.1524153

89. Mohanan, S., Tapp, H., McWilliams, A., Dulin, M. (2014). Obesity and asthma: Pathophysiology and implications for diagnosis and management in primary care. *Experimental Biology and Medicine (Maywood)*, 239(11), 1531–1540. DOI: 10.1177/1535370214525302

90. Mongraw-Chaffin M, Foster, M.C., Anderson, C.A.M., et al. (2018). Metabolically Healthy Obesity, Transition to Metabolic Syndrome, and Cardiovascular Risk. *Journal of the American College of Cardiology*, 71(17), 1857-1865. DOI: 10.1016/j.jacc.2018.02.055

91. Muktabhant, B., Lawrie, T.A., Lumbiganon, P., Laopaiboon, M. (2015). Diet or exercise, or both, for preventing excessive weight gain in pregnancy. *The Cochrane Database of Systematic Reviews,* Jun 15;(6):CD007145. DOI: 10.1002/14651858.CD007145.pub3

92. National Institute of Diabetes and Digestive and Kidney Diseases. (2016). Prescription Medications to Treat Overweight and Obesity. https://www.niddk.nih.gov/health-information/weight-management/prescription-medications-treat-overweight-obesity

93. National Heart, Lung, and Blood Institute. Guide to Behavior Change. Your Weight Is Important. https://www.nhlbi.nih.gov/health/educational/lose_wt/behavior.htm

94. National Heart, Lung, and Blood Institute. Heart Failure. https://www.nhlbi.nih.gov/health-topics/heart-failure

95. National Institute of Diabetes and Digestive and Kidney Diseases. (2017). Overweight & Obesity Statistics. https://www.niddk.nih.gov/health-information/health-statistics/overweight-obesity

96. Neogi, T. (2011). Gout. *New England Journal of Medicine*, 364(5), 443-452. DOI: 10.1056/NEJMcp1001124

97. Orloff, N.C., Flammer, A., Hartnett, J., et al. (2016). Food cravings in pregnancy: Preliminary evidence for a role in excess gestational weight gain. *Appetite*, 105, 259-265. DOI: 10.1016/j.appet.2016.04.040

98. Ouakinin, S.R.S., Barreira, D.P., Gois, C.J. (2018). Depression and Obesity: Integrating the Role of Stress, Neuroendocrine Dysfunction and Inflammatory Pathways. *Frontiers in Endocrinology (Lausanne)*, 9, 431. DOI: 10.3389/fendo.2018.00431

99. Pandey, A., LaMonte, M., Klein, L., et al. (2017). Relationship Between Physical Activity, Body Mass Index, and Risk of Heart Failure. *Journal of the American College of Cardiology*, 69(9), 1129-1142. DOI: 10.1016/j.jacc.2016.11.081

100. Patnode, C.D., Evans, C.V., Senger, C.A., et al. (2017). Behavioral Counseling to Promote a Healthful Diet and Physical Activity for Cardiovascular Disease Prevention in Adults Without Known Cardiovascular Disease Risk Factors: Updated Systematic Review for the U.S. Preventive Services Task Force [Internet]. Rockville (MD): Agency for Healthcare Research and Quality (US). U.S. Preventive Services Task Force Evidence Syntheses, Report No.: 15-05222-EF-1.

101. Rao, V.N., Zhao, D., Allison, M.A., et al. (2018). Adiposity and Incident Heart Failure and its Subtypes: MESA (Multi-Ethnic Study of Atherosclerosis). *JACC Heart Failure,* pii: S2213-1779(18)30559-6. DOI: 10.1016/j.jchf.2018.07.009

102. Rebello, C.J., Greenway, F.L. (2016), Reward-Induced Eating: Therapeutic Approaches to Addressing Food Cravings. *Advances in Therapy*, 33(11), 1853-1866.

103. Rehm, C.D., Peñalvo, J.L., Afshin, A., Mozaffarian, D. (2016). Dietary Intake Among US Adults, 1999-2012. *Journal* of the American Medical Association, 315(23), 2542-2553. DOI: 10.1001/jama.2016.7491

104. Roberge, J.B., Van Hulst, A., Barnett, T.A., et al. (2018). Lifestyle Habits, Dietary Factors, and the Metabolically Unhealthy Obese Phenotype in Youth. *The Journal of Pediatrics*, Oct 23. pii: S0022-3476(18)31237-X. DOI: 10.1016/j.jpeds.2018.08.063

105. Romagnolo, D.F., Selmin, O.I. (2017). Mediterranean Diet and Prevention of Chronic Diseases. *Nutrition Today*, 52(5), 208-222. DOI: 10.1097/NT.0000000000000228.

106. Romero-Corral, A., Caples, S.M., Lopez-Jimenez, F., et al. (2010). Interactions Between Obesity and Obstructive Sleep Apnea. Implications for Treatment. *Chest*, 137(3), 711–719. DOI: 10.1378/chest.09-0360

107. Rosen, C.L. (2011). Clinical practice. Vitamin D Insufficiency. *New England Journal of Medicine*, 364(3), 248-254. DOI: 10.1056/NEJMcp1009570

108. Rosenbaum, D.L., White, K.S. (2015). The relation of anxiety, depression, and stress to binge eating behavior. *Journal of Health Psychology*, 20(6), 887-898. DOI: 10.1177/1359105315580212

109. Russo, C., Jin, Z., Homma, S., et al. (2011). Effect of obesity and overweight on left ventricular diastolic function: A community-based study in an elderly cohort. *Journal of the American College of Cardiology*, 57(12, 1368-1374. DOI: 10.1016/j.jacc.2010.10.042

110. The Quote Garden. (2016). Quotations about Dieting & Weight Loss. http://www.quotegarden.com/dieting.html

111. Saito H, Kimura, Y., Tashima, S., et al. (2009). Psychological factors that promote behavior modification by obese patients. *BioPsychoSocial Medicine*, 3(9). DOI: 10.1186/1759-0759-3-9

112. Sampath, K., Rothstein, R.I. (2017). Selected Endoscopic Gastric Devices for Obesity. *Gastrointestinal Endoscopy Clinics of North America*, 27(2), 267-275. DOI: 10.1016/j.giec.2017.01.005

113. Saunders, K.H., Igel, L.I., Saumoy, M., et al. (2018). Devices and Endoscopic Bariatric Therapies for Obesity. *Current Obesity Reports*, 7(2), 162-171. DOI: 10.1007/s13679-018-0307-x

114. Saunders, K.H., Igel, L.I., Shukla, A.P., Aronne, L.J. (2016). Drug-induced weight gain: Rethinking our choices. *Journal of Family Practice*, 65(11), 780-788.

115. Saunders, K.H., Umashanker, D., Igel, L.I., et al. (2018). Obesity Pharmacotherapy. *The Medical Clinics of North America*, 102(1), 135-148. DOI: 10.1016/j.mcna.2017.08.010

116. Schauer, P.B., Bhatt, D.L., Kirwan, J.P., et al. (2017). Bariatric surgery versus intensive medical therapy for diabetes—5-year outcomes. *New England Journal of Medicine*, 376(7), 641-651.

117. Schulte, E.M., Grilo, C.M., Gearhardt, A.N. (2016). Shared and unique mechanisms underlying binge eating disorder and addictive disorders. *Clinical Psychology Review*, 44, 125-139. DOI: 10.1016/j.cpr.2016.02.001

REFERENCES

118. Sinha, R. (2018). Role of addiction and stress neurobiology on food intake and obesity. *Biological Psychology*, 131, 5-13. DOI: 10.1016/j.biopsycho.2017.05.001

119. Sleep for Kids. "Children, Obesity, and Sleep." http://www.sleepforkids.org/html/obesity.html

120. Smithson, E.F., Hill, A.J. (2017). It is not how much you crave but what you do with it that counts: behavioural responses to foodcraving during weight management. *European Journal or Clinical Nutrition*, 71(5), 625-630. DOI: 10.1038/ejcn.2016.235

121. Spaeth, A.M., Dinges, D.F., Goel, N. (2017). Objective Measurements of Energy Balance Are Associated With Sleep Architecture in Healthy Adults. *Sleep*, 40(1), DOI: 10.1093/sleep/zsw018

122. Srivastava, G. Apovian, C. (2018). Future Pharmacotherapy for Obesity: New Anti-obesity Drugs on the Horizon. *Current Obesity Reports*, 7(2), 147-161. DOI: 10.1007/s13679-018-0300-4

123. Stevenson, B.L., Dvorak, R.D., Wonderlich, S.A., et al. (2018). Emotions before and after loss of control eating. *Eating Disorders*, 26(6), 505-522. DOI: 10.1080/10640266.2018.1453634

124. Strazzullo, P., D'Elia, L., Cairella, G., et al. (2010). Excess body weight and incidence of stroke: meta-analysis of prospective studies with 2 million participants. *Stroke*, 41(5), e418-26. DOI: 10.1161/STROKEAHA.109.576967

125. Suliga, E., Cieśla, E., Rębak, D, et al. (2018). Relationship Between Sitting Time, Physical Activity, and Metabolic Syndrome Among Adults Depending on Body Mass Index (BMI). *Medical Science Monitor*, 24, 7633-7645. DOI: 10.12659/MSM.907582

126. Sumithran, P., Prendergast, L.A., Dellridge, E., et al. (2011). Long-term persistence of hormonal adaptations to weight loss. *New England Journal of Medicine*, 365(17), 1597-1604. DOI: 10.1056/NEJMoa1105816

127. Taler, S.J.(2018). Initial treatment of hypertension. *New England Journal of Medicine*, 378(7), 636-644. DOI: 10.1056/NEJMcp1613481

128. Tapper, K., Turner, A. (2018). The effect of a mindfulness-based decentering strategy on chocolate craving. *Appetite*, 130, 157-162. DOI: 10.1016/j.appet.2018.08.011

129. Tapper, K. (2018). Mindfulness and craving: effects and mechanisms. Clinical Psychology Review, 59, 101-117. DOI: 10.1016/j.cpr.2017.11.003

130. Tate, C.M., Geliebter, A. (2017). Intragastric Balloon Treatment for Obesity: Review of Recent Studies. *Advances in Therapy*, 34(8), 1859-1875. DOI: 10.1007/s12325-017-0562-3

131. Thangaratinam, S, Rogozińska, E., Jolly, K., et al. (2012). Interventions to reduce or prevent obesity in pregnant women: a systematic review. *Health Technology Assessment*, 16(31):iii-iv, 1-191. DOI: 10.3310/hta16310

132. Thorpe, K.E., Yang, Z., Long, K.M., Garvey, W.T. (2013). The impact of weight loss among seniors on Medicare spending. *Health Economics Review*, 3(1), 7. DOI: 10.1186/2191-1991-3-7

133. Tian, H., Guo, X., Wang, X., et al. (2013). Chromium picolinate supplementation for overweight or obese adults. *The Cochrane Database of Systematic Reviews*, (11):CD010063. DOI: 10.1002/14651858.CD010063.pub2

134. Tuomilehto, H., Seppä, J, Uusitupa, M. (2013). Obesity and obstructive sleep apnea--clinical significance of weight loss. *Sleep Medicine Reviews*, 17(5), 321-329. DOI: 10.1016/j.smrv.2012.08.002

135. Ulrik, C.S.. (2016). Asthma and obesity: is weight reduction the key to achieve asthma control? *Current Opinion in Pulmonary Medicine*, 22(1), 69-73. DOI: 10.1097/MCP.0000000000000226

136. Vander Wal, J.S. (2012). Night eating syndrome: a critical review of the literature. *Clinical Psychology Review*, 32(1), 49-59. DOI: 10.1016/j.cpr.2011.11.001

137. Van Horn, L. (2014). A diet by any other name is still about energy. *Journal of the American Medical Association*, 312(9), 900-901. DOI: 10.1001/jama.2014.10837

138. van Strien, T. (2018). Causes of Emotional Eating and Matched Treatment of Obesity. *Current Diabetes Reports*, 18(6), 35. DOI: 10.1007/s11892-018-1000-x

139. van Strien, T., Konttinen, H., Homberg, J.R., et al. (2016). Emotional eating as a mediator between depression and weight gain. *Appetite*, 100, 216-224. DOI: 10.1016/j.appet.2016.02.034

140. Vargas, E.J., Rizk, M., Bazerbachi, F., Abu Dayyeh, B.K. (2018). Medical Devices for Obesity Treatment: Endoscopic Bariatric Therapies. *Medical Clinics of North America*, 102(1), 149-163. DOI: 10.1016/j.mcna.2017.08.013

141. Verzijl, C.L., Ahlich, E., Schlauch, R.C., Rancourt, D. (2018). The role of craving in emotional and uncontrolled eating. *Appetite*, 123, 146-151. DOI: 10.1016/j.appet.2017.12.014

142. Vyas, D., Deshpande, K., Pandya, Y. (2017). Advances in endoscopic balloon therapy for weight loss and its limitations. *World Journal of Gastroenterology*, 23(44), 7813-7817. DOI: 10.3748/wjg.v23.i44.7813

143. Wharton, S. Raiber, L., Serodio, K.J., et al. (2018). Medications that cause weight gain and alternatives in Canada: a narrative review. *Diabetes, Metabolic Syndrome and Obesity: Targets and Therapy*,11, 427-438. DOI: 10.2147/DMSO.S171365

144. Win, S., Parakh, K., Eze-Nliam, C.M., et al. (2011). Depressive symptoms, physical inactivity, and risk of cardiovascular mortality in older adults: the Cardiovascular Health Study. *Heart,* 97(6): 500-505. DOI: 10.1136/hrt.2010.209767

145. Wurtman, J, Wurtman, R. (2018). The Trajectory from Mood to Obesity. *Current Obesity Reports*, 7(1), 1-5. DOI: 10.1007/s13679-017-0291-6

146. Yanovski, S.Z., Yanovski, J.A. (2014). Long-term drug treatment for obesity: a systematic and clinical review. *Journal of the American Medical Association*, 311(1), 74-86. DOI: 10.1001/jama.2013.281361

147. Yeh, G.Y., McCarthy, E.P., Wayne, P.M., et al. (2011). Tai chi exercise in patients with chronic heart failure: A randomized clinical trial. *Archives of Internal Medicine,* 171(8), 750-757. DOI: 10.1001/archinternmed.2011.150

148. Yu, W. (011). A losing personality: the slimming effect of being neurotic. *Scientific American Mind,* January, 60-63.

149. Zimberg, I.Z., Dâmaso, A., Del Re, M., (2012). Short sleep duration and obesity: mechanisms and future perspectives. *Cell Biochemistry and Function*, 30(6), 524-529. DOI: 10.1002/cbf.2832

GLOSSARY

ACE (angiotensin converting enzyme)Inhibitors are drugs that lower blood pressure by decreasing the activity of the angiotensin-converting enzyme.

Amphetamines are drugs known to stimulate the central nervous system. Derivatives of amphetamines are used to treat Attention Deficit Hyperactivity Disorder. A known side-effect of amphetamines is appetite suppression.

Anorexia Nervosa is a problematic eating disorder affecting mostly younger women. It is characterized as a fear of weight gain and leads to significant unhealthy and potentially life-threatening weight loss.

Ayurveda the word Ayurveda means "the knowledge of life" in Sanskrit. Ayurveda is a holistic and herbal medical approach based on 5000 years of traditional Hindu medicine.

Benzodiazepines are psychoactive drugs that act as tranquilizers. These drugs are used to treat insomnia and anxiety. Caution is warranted because of their addictive properties.

Biliopancreatic Diversion is a form of weight-loss surgery in which part of the stomach is either removed or made unavailable. The upper duodenum is bypassed, and the remaining stomach pouch is attached to the lower duodenum, decreasing nutrient absorption and leading to weight loss.

Binge Eating is a condition in which a person eats large amounts of food in a short time. Episodes of binge eating may be separated by periods of fasting.

BMI (body mass index) is the weight in kilograms divided by the square of the person's height in meters. BMI is often used as a measure of overweight or obesity.

GLOSSARY

Bulimia Nervosa is a very serious eating disorder that affects mostly women. It is characterized by compulsive overeating (binge eating), followed by purging with induced vomiting, use of laxatives and/or diuretics.

Chitosan is a natural polymer made from the chitin of crustacean shells. Chitosan is a string of glucosamine molecules, and is used as a weight-loss aid to bind fats in the digestive tract.

Cholecystokinin is a hormone secreted by the small intestine that stimulates the release of pancreatic enzymes which digest dietary fats.

Chromium is an essential mineral involved with glucose metabolism. Chromium deficiency may result in impaired glucose tolerance and peripheral neuropathy (numbness, or tingling sensations in fingers or feet, for example).

Chronic Fatigue Syndrome is a condition that includes symptoms of fatigue lasting over 6 months not relieved by rest and multiple somatic symptoms. The causes of chronic fatigue syndrome include genetic predisposition, neuro-endocrine dysfunction, multiple viruses, and environmental factors.

Ciliary Neurotrophic Factor is a compound that causes loss of appetite and weight loss. However, when recombinant ciliary neurotrophic factor was used in human clinical trials, its efficacy was inhibited because clinical trial patients formed antibodies to the recombinant protein.

Circadian Rhythm is a cycling 24-hr biological clock that regulates sleep and eating patterns. In humans, disruption of circadian rhythm results in a disturbed release of melatonin, and sleep disorders.

CLA (conjugated linoleic acid) is an omega-6 fatty acid derived from dairy and meat fat, and is thought to have anti-cancer and weight loss properties. Its weight loss and anti-cancer benefits have not yet been clinically proven in controlled human studies.

Cognitive Behavioral Therapy is a combination of two effective types of psychotherapy; cognitive and behavioral. Its focus is to change a person's thoughts or cognitive patterns, which in turn will alter behavior patterns and emotions. It is heavily focused on solving problems.

Cortisol is a hormone released by the adrenal gland as a response to stress. Prolonged cortisol release can increase blood glucose and blood pressure, cause weight gain and suppress the immune system. A product of cortisol is hydrocortisone, which is used to treat rheumatoid arthritis, allergic reactions, and many autoimmune disorders.

CPAP (continuous positive airway pressure) CPAP devices are used by individuals who have sleep apnea to keep the nasal and throat passages open, prevent snoring and improve sleep quality.

C Reactive Protein is a protein found in blood that increases in response to inflammation. Elevated C reactive protein levels can be found in heart attack patients and in patients who have connective tissue diseases, rheumatoid arthritis, lupus, cancer, infections, obesity, and smoking.

Cushing's Disease is a syndrome caused by excess corticosteroid secretion from the adrenal glands, leading to central obesity and muscle weakness, high blood pressure, high blood sugar, abdominal striae and "buffalo hump" between the shoulder blades.

Diabetes, type 1 otherwise known as "insulin-dependent diabetes," is a disease in which patients are not able to produce insulin and have high blood sugar as a result. It is typically diagnosed in children and teens.

Diabetes, type 2 otherwise known as "non-insulin-dependent diabetes", also formerly known as "adult-onset diabetes" is a condition in which an individual may produce decreased amounts of insulin or may be resistant to the effects of insulin, and as a result, develops high blood sugar. Complications include nephropathy, neuropathy, retinopathy, and vascular disease.

Dopamine is a neurotransmitter in the brain that affects muscle movement, healthy mood, mental function, alertness, and the ability to experience pleasure. Dopamine deficiency results in Parkinson's Disease.

Dumping Syndrome also called rapid gastric emptying, results in nausea, vomiting, and diarrhea due to large amounts of undigested food in the small intestine. It is common in patients who have undergone gastric bypass.

Endorphins are naturally-occurring opiates produced in the brain in response to strenuous exercise. Endorphins also decrease the response to pain.

Ephedra is a stimulant derived from the Ma Huang plant (a Chinese herb) that was formerly used as an appetite suppressant. Ephedra also increases blood pressure and can cause heart attacks, strokes, and increase the risk of heat stroke in athletes.

Epidemic is defined as disease affecting unexpected or large numbers of individuals in a short period of time.

Fibromyalgia is a syndrome characterized by generalized muscle pain and stiffness. In addition, the patient must exhibit pain sensitivity in 11 of 18 designated tender points. Sleep architecture is usually abnormal.

Galanin is a hormone secreted by the hypothalamus. It increases before growth spurts in teenagers. When injected, galanin causes increased fat intake.

Gastroplasty is a surgical procedure for obesity in which the stomach volume is reduced using staples or a band in order to decrease food consumption, providing a feeling of fullness, and aid weight loss.

Genotype is the specific genetic makeup of an individual.

Ghrelin is a hormone secreted by gasric cells before a meal. Ghrelin increases appetite by acting on the hypothalamus.

Glucorticoids are hormones secreted by the adrenal glands that can cause the liver to produce glucose from protein and fat. A common glucocorticoid is cortisol. Hydrocortisone, related to cortisol, is used to treat certain inflammatory conditions, such as asthma, allergic reactions, rheumatoid arthritis, and numerous autoimmune disorders.

Glycemic Index is a nutritional scale that ranks carbohydrates according to how much and how quickly glucose is released after consumption. A high glycemic index results from ingestion of simple sugars, quick absorption, and a rapid glucose spike. Low glycemic index foods are generally complex carbohydrates that are slowly absorbed in the digestive tract with a more balanced glucose release. They can be helpful in weight loss.

Growth Hormone is secreted by the pituitary gland and affects bone and muscle growth, and fat, protein and carbohydrate metabolism.

HDL (high density lipoprotein) is a molecule that binds to cholesterol and takes it to the liver to be metabolized. High HDL levels are important for cardiovascular health.

Hydroxycitrate a substance derived from the Garcinia Cambogia plant is included in several weight-loss products. It is thought to increase fat metabolism and decrease appetite. However, these findings have not been conclusively proven in human clinical trials.

Hypnotics are drugs used as sedatives to relieve insomnia and anxiety.

Hypothyroidism is a condition in which the thyroid does not make enough thyroid hormone. Thyroid hormone is used by the body to regulate metabolism. Symptoms include weight gain, fatigue, lethargy, constipation, dry skin, cold intolerance, brittle hair and nails.

Hypoparathyroidism is a condition in which the parathyroid glands do not release enough parathyroid hormone, resulting in calcium deficiency and numerous physical symptoms, which can include tetany.

Impaired Glucose Tolerance is considered by some to be a precursor to Type 2 diabetes. It is diagnosed using a Glucose tolerance test, and defined as a 2-hr glucose value range of 140 – 199 mg/dL after a 75 g glucose challenge.

Insulin is a hormone produced by the pancreas that promotes glucose utilization and protein synthesis.

Insulin-like Growth Factor is very similar in structure to insulin. It is produced by the liver in response to Growth Hormone to regulate cell growth and differentiation in several areas, such as bone, nerves, skin, lungs, and muscle.

Insulin Resistance is a condition in which the insulin receptors in the body are insensitive to insulin, resulting in impaired glucose metabolism.

Intestinal Bypass was initially used to treat morbid obesity. In this procedure, large segments of the small intestine are bypassed, leaving a reduced absorptive surface, resulting in weight loss. However, the procedure is no longer used due to numerous side effects.

Ketosis is the presence of abnormally high blood levels of acidic substances called ketones. These substances are produced when fat is broken down in the liver and converted to energy. Ketones can suppress appetite.

Laparoscopic Gastric Banding used for long term weight loss in obese individuals, is a procedure in which a band is placed around the stomach. Placement of this band allows an obese person to feel full after eating only a small portion and thus enables him or her to lose weight.

LDL (low density lipoproteins) transport cholesterol in the bloodstream. As LDL carries cholesterol into the arteries, high levels of this lipoprotein have been associated with atherosclerosis, myocardial infarctions, strokes and peripheral vascular disease.

Leptin is a hormone that is produced by fat cells; it plays a key role in metabolism and the regulation of adipose tissue. It appears to be involved in regulating food intake and fat storage in the body by acting on the hypothalamus.

MC4R Deficiency the melanocortin-4 receptor (MC4R) is a 332-amino acid protein that plays a role in metabolic regulation and energy intake through a pathway involving leptin. Mutations in the MC4R gene cause increased food intake and obesity, which develop in infancy and childhood.

Melatonin is a hormone that is derived from serotonin and released by the pineal gland. It plays a role in sleep, aging, and reproduction in mammals.

Metabolic Syndrome also known as Syndrome X, metabolic syndrome is a cluster of medical conditions that occur together, which increase the risk of cardiovascular disease, stroke and diabetes mellitus. These conditions include increased blood pressure, elevated insulin levels, excess body fat around the waist and abnormal cholesterol levels.

GLOSSARY

Multiple Sclerosis is a chronic degenerative disorder of the nervous system, characterized by the gradual destruction of myelin, the fatty covering that insulates axons in the brain and spinal cord. Myelin facilitates the transmission of electrochemical messages between the brain, the spinal cord, and the rest of the body, and when it becomes damaged, transmission may be delayed or blocked completely. Symptoms of multiple sclerosis include muscular weakness, loss of coordination, and speech and visual disturbances.

Natural Killer Cells also known as NK cells, K cells, and killer cells, are a type of lymphocyte and a component of the body's immune system. These cells do not destroy invading pathogens directly but rather attack infected cells and possible cancerous cells through a process called antibody-dependent cell-mediated cytotoxicity.

Nephropathy is an abnormal state involving the kidney, usually associated with or secondary to a pathological process such as diabetes

Neuropeptide Y is a 36-amino acid peptide neurotransmitter found in the brain and autonomic nervous system. It has been associated with a number of physiologic processes in the brain, including the regulation of energy balance and appetite, memory and learning, and epilepsy. Neuropeptide Y can intensify cravings for carbohydrate-rich foods.

Norepinephrine also known as noradrenalin, is both a hormone and a neurotransmitter and is secreted by the adrenal glands and the nerve endings of the sympathetic nervous system. Its release causes a number of physiologic effects, including vasoconstriction, and increases in heart rate, blood pressure, and glucose levels. Norepinephrine can trigger the desire for carbohydrates.

NSAIDs (nonsteroidal anti-inflammatory drugs) include drugs such as aspirin, ibuprofen, naproxen and others. These are medications that possess analgesic, antipyretic and anti-inflammatory properties, and the term non-steroidal is used to distinguish them from steroids.

Opiates is a broad term used to describe any one of various sedative narcotics that contain opium, or one or more of its natural or synthetic derivatives.

Pandemic is an epidemic that occurs over a wide geographic area, and affects a large proportion of the population.

Pineal Gland also called the pineal body and pineal organ, it is a small, cone-shaped organ located near the center of the brain that secretes the hormone melatonin.

Polycystic Ovary Syndrome is a disorder of the ovaries, characterized by hirsutism, obesity, menstrual abnormalities, infertility, and enlarged ovaries. Also called Stein-Leventhal syndrome, it is usually caused by an elevated level of luteinizing hormone, androgen, or estrogen that may result in an abnormal cycle of gonadotropin release by the pituitary gland.

Polysomnogram is a record of the physiologic variables that occur during sleep, as obtained by continuous monitoring. This test is used to diagnose many types of sleep disorders, including narcolepsy and sleep apnea, and entails the simultaneous recording of the electrical activity of the brain, eye movements, skeletal muscle activation, and heart rhythm.

POMC Deficiency Proopiomelanocortin (POMC) is the precursor for pituitary adrenocorticotropic hormone (ACTH), which is essential for maintaining adrenal cortical function. POMC is part of the central melanocortin system, which plays a key role in regulating appetite and energy. A genetic POMC deficiency syndrome has been described in humans, and is characterized by severe early-onset obesity.

GLOSSARY

Prader-Willi Syndrome is a congenital syndrome characterized by short stature, mental retardation, and excessive eating and obesity. The syndrome was first described in 1956 by Swiss pediatricians Andrea Prader and Heinrich Willi.

PTSD (Post-Traumatic Stress Disorder) is an anxiety disorder also known as delayed-stress disorder, delayed-stress syndrome, and post-traumatic stress syndrome. This disorder primarily affects individuals who have experienced or witnessed profoundly traumatic events, such as torture, murder, rape, or wartime combat. It is characterized by recurrent flashbacks of the traumatic event, recurrent nightmares, depression, irritability, anxiety, fatigue, forgetfulness, and social withdrawal.

Retinopathy is a term used to describe any number of noninflammatory degenerative disorders of the retina, including those which may cause blindness. It is also caused by diabetes.

Roux-En-Y Gastric Bypass is a procedure almost exclusively used in surgical weight-loss applications to correct morbid obesity. It reduces the capacity of the stomach by creating a smaller stomach pouch, which can only hold about one ounce of fluid. In the procedure, the surgeon also constructs a tiny stomach outlet, which causes food to leave the stomach more slowly.

Sarcopenia can be defined as the age-related loss of muscle mass, strength and function. It strongly influences strength and mobility, and is a factor in the development of frailty and likelihood of falls and fractures in the elderly.

Seasonal Affective Disorder is a depressive disorder associated with the reduction of daylight during the shorter days of late autumn and winter. Symptoms include loss of energy and sexual drive, restlessness, and sometimes a craving for carbohydrates.

Serotonin is a neurotransmitter synthesized from the amino acid tryptophan. It plays an important role in the biochemistry of depression, migraine, bipolar disorder and anxiety, and may also have some effect on sexuality, appetite, and pain

Set Point Theory is a theory that every person has a personal metabolic rate, which helps maintain a certain weight, regardless of calorie intake. This personal weight or set point is believed to be the reason why many individuals find that they reach weight loss plateaus, or that they keep regaining lost weight.

Sleep Apnea is a sleep disorder characterized by periodic and temporary cessations of breathing that occur during sleep. It is usually caused by an obstruction of the upper airway, and often affects individuals who are overweight. In a small number of people, sleep apnea is cause by a neurologic disorder that creates a disturbance in the brain's respiratory center. Daytime somnolence, irritability, morning headaches, and difficulty with learning and memory are common symptoms.

SSRIs (selective serotonin reuptake inhibitors) are a class of drugs that inhibit the uptake of serotonin by neurons of the central nervous system. These medications are used primarily to treat depression, obsessive compulsive disorder, anxiety, and PMS.

Triglycerides are fatty compounds that circulate in the bloodstream and are stored in adipose tissue. They consist of three molecules of fatty acid combined with a molecule of the alcohol glycerol, and form the backbone of many types of fats. High triglyceride levels are a risk factor for heart disease.

Tryptophan is an essential amino acid that is necessary for normal growth and development, and is the precursor of several substances, including serotonin and niacin. Foods containing tryptophan are thought to enhance relaxation and sleep.

1. T
2. F
3 T

4)

5.

6 - D

7 -

8 -

9 - D

10 - A

11 -

12

13 -

14 - C

15 -

16 -

17 - B

18 -

19 -

20 -

21 -

22 -

23 -

24 -

25 -

26 -

27 -

28 -

29 -

30 -